> *"To be in excellent physical condition is a great feeling. It changes my entire outlook on what I think I can accomplish, both on and off the field. Once you are in shape, everything else is relatively easy. You are functioning on all cylinders and can concentrate on the mental demands of your game."*
>
> —CARL BANKS

Getting in good shape takes more than simply exercise. It takes proper nutrition, fitness, and a positive mental attitude. This comprehensive guide has information on it all. And interwoven with the program are fascinating anecdotes and Banks' commentary on classic games and plays. And exciting action photographs show Banks doing what he does best. The devoted Giants linebacker also maintains a powerful anti-drug message throughout, which makes this guide not only entertaining but timely and important for the young player in any game.

CARL BANKS, two-time Super Bowl veteran, is an all-pro star linebacker for the New York Giants. *Sports Illustrated* called Banks' 1987 season "one of the finest years any defensive player has ever had." MICHAEL EISEN is a Giants beat writer for the *Newark Star Ledger*.

D1225976

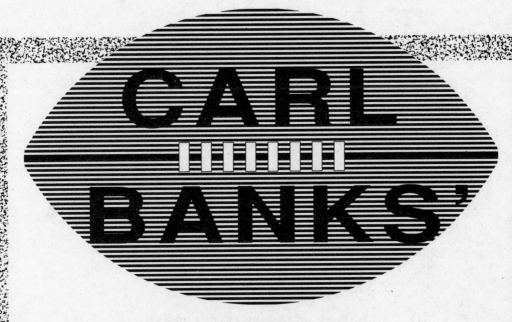

FOOTBALL
TRAINING PROGRAM

A Conditioning and Total Health Program
for the Young Athlete

CARL BANKS
WITH MICHAEL EISEN

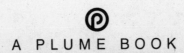

A PLUME BOOK

PLUME
Published by the Penguin Group
Penguin Books USA Inc., 375 Hudson Street,
New York, New York 10014, U.S.A.
Penguin Books Ltd, 27 Wrights Lane,
London W8 5TZ, England
Penguin Books Australia Ltd, Ringwood,
Victoria, Australia
Penguin Books Canada Ltd, 2801 John Street,
Markham, Ontario, Canada L3R 1B4
Penguin Books (N.Z.) Ltd, 182–190 Wairau Road,
Auckland 10, New Zealand

Penguin Books Ltd, Registered Offices:
Harmondsworth, Middlesex, England

First published by Plume, an imprint of New American Library,
a division of Penguin Books USA Inc.

First Printing, June 1991
10 9 8 7 6 5 4 3 2 1

 REGISTERED TRADEMARK—MARCA REGISTRADA

Library of Congress Cataloging-in-Publication Data

Banks, Carl.
    Carl Banks' conditioning and total health program / Carl Banks ;
with Michael Eisen.
        p.   cm.
    ISBN 0-452-26620-3
    1. Football—Training. 2. Physical fitness. 3. Youth—Health and
hygiene. 4. Youth—Nutrition. I. Eisen, Michael. II. Title.
GV953.5.B36   1991
796.332'07—dc20   90-25797
                                                           CIP

Printed in the United States of America
Set in Aster
Designed by Stanley S. Drate/Folio Graphics Co. Inc.

For Karen,
whose love, patience and understanding
I could not live without.

Michael Eisen

Carl Banks' Acknowledgments

First and foremost, I want to thank God for giving me the ability to succeed at football.

Thanks also go to Mom and Dad for allowing me to participate and for insisting that I wear my cup (smile, Dad) as well as the proper equipment; to Rosey Haywood for my beginning and for telling me, "This is where it's at"; and to my wonderful wife, Cheryl, and our beautiful daughter, Carla, for their unselfish love and for putting up with my many moods during the season—you mean the world to me; keep feeding me those healthy meals. Thanks to my junior high school coaches for believing in me when my talent was poor and the competition was tough; and to Freddie Spence for finding me when they said I wasn't good enough. My special thanks go to Moses "Cudd" Lacy—I owe it all to you. You taught me the value of conditioning and the values a true athlete must have. You made me understand the meaning of toughness, both mental and physical. Because of what you taught me, I will never be able to accept defeat. You taught me that publicity is like poison: as long as it's left in its proper place, it won't harm you, but as soon as it's ingested, it can kill you. I love you and thank you for making me a football player instead of just a linebacker. Special thanks go to Lonnie Young, for getting me through the tough times, for pushing me during our workouts, for teaching me how to run for speed, and for reinforcing the teachings of Coach Lacy. We've made it together and as long as we keep our heads on straight, we will keep that edge that everyone wants to know about. The blood, sweat, tears, and arguments—I love you for them all. A big thank-you also to Tim Cunningham, for all that jazz; to Ray Taylor, Ty Willingham, and Sherm Lewis; to Curt Shattenhiemer, for not making me a tight end at Michigan State; to Clarence Underwood; and to Mary Kay and Pam and all my friends at Beecher High School and in the Flint area.

CONTENTS

FOREWORD

by Ronnie Barnes,
Head Trainer, New York Giants

Carl Banks works as hard in the off-season as he does during the football season, which this workout program demonstrates very clearly. He works hard all year round. That's important to him. When he's not at Giants Stadium, he's working. That is certifiable by the success he has had in his career.

In sports medicine, we know that the best way to prevent athletic injuries is through year-round conditioning and a proper flexibility program, as well as a conditioning program that enhances cardiovascular endurance and strength. Carl's program includes all of these elements. It's one reason his program has been such a big part of his success.

We have found that athletes who don't condition themselves year-round—such as football players who play in the fall and don't do anything else in the off-season—are the players injured most frequently and those most likely to look for quick fixes to get back into shape, such as starvation diets prior to training camp or steroids to make them bigger. None of these are really very ethical nor very sound practices. Many are extremely unhealthy.

Carl has avoided these shortcuts and taken the scientific approach, a process by which one can prepare himself for any sports endeavor in which he wants to participate. It includes a proper warm-up and exercises for conditioning, flexibility, cardiovascular endurance, and strength. Carl has all of these elements in his program.

The principles of conditioning that Carl details in this book, including warm-up, stretching, strength, and his general exercise protocol, are those that I would strongly recommend for young athletes who are looking for a program that can help them get into condition. This program will get you going in the right direction and will set you on winning ways. Carl used these conditioning principles to help develop himself into a premier linebacker.

Carl understands the importance of nutrition and monitors his diet. Two things are vital for him to maintain an optimal level of performance. One is that he be as fit as possible, which can be determined by the percentage of body fat. On a regular basis, we measure the players' body fat. Carl has always had one of the lowest percentages of body fat on the Giants. He has maintained it through his vigorous exercise program, as well as a reduction of fat and an increase in carbohydrates in his diet. We know that that combination is the best for peak performance.

The second aspect of Carl's healthy diet is his living a clean life. It has been said that what athletes eat and drink is reflected in their performance. The use of alcohol and drugs lowers your performance level and threatens your life which is why Carl has made a point of not using either. He doesn't smoke, doesn't use alcohol, and gets proper rest. That's all part of the reason for his success.

The rules for athletes have not changed. Twenty years ago we told athletes not to smoke because it reduces cardiovascular endurance. We told them that alcohol is bad, that it decreases your reflexes and increases the amount of fat in your body. Those rules for clean living haven't changed. Carl has followed those rules and they have helped him to be an outstanding football player.

Carl has always wanted to know what he could do to make himself better. When he has an injury he comes into my office and he wants a checklist. He says, "Write down everything I need to do to get better." If he has to do 50 leg extensions and 50 leg curls and ride the exercise bike, I write it all down so he can do it.

He takes the same approach with nutrition. We have a nutrition computer in the training room, which lists all the calories and target food groups the players should be aware of. Early in his career, Carl kept a diary of what he was eating and counted up all the calories. He found that he was on the right track.

Carl is deeply saddened and upset when he finds out that someone on his team is taking a shortcut. When Lawrence Taylor was suspended for drug use, Carl was devastated. He came to me and said, "Ronnie, why can't he control himself? Why does he let this happen?" He felt that Lawrence was letting his team down, and more important, he felt that Lawrence was letting himself down, and he just couldn't understand it.

We talked about addiction and what it does. I think both the personal crisis that Lawrence has gone through and what Carl has seen in the NFL and on our team has given him the impetus to want to help other people.

Carl is a good student of the game. He reads a lot and asks a lot of questions about what he has to do to improve. He will read an article about nutrition or conditioning or substance abuse and he'll ask the doctor or me about something he may not understand. I'm never sure whether he wants to know for himself or whether he's using it to help other players. Carl is the kind of guy who passes the knowledge on to other individuals.

I think Carl sees himself as the next leader of this team. I think he already is, by virtue of his play, his life-style and clean living, and his genuine interest in people. And, I think he wants to be ready to help both younger and older players with whatever interests them or bothers them.

Carl leads by example. A lot of people have read the novels about pro football, which emphasize wine, women, and song. But the new breed of football players, though we have our exceptions, are students of the game. They're committed to excellence and being the very best they can be.

There are some things we learn early on that we know help lead to success in athletics. They include dedication, sacrifice, hard work, honesty, loyalty, 100 percent commitment to the game, respect for your opponent, and preparation. They are all components Carl learned early in his athletic career. They helped him become a great athlete; he still works as hard as he ever did.

He is tremendously inspired by successful athletes. He knows Magic Johnson and some successful boxers. Carl knows he's going to work as hard as he can to be the very best athlete, the very best football player, the very best linebacker, and the very best Giant he can be.

INTRODUCTION

by Bill Belichick
Head Coach, Cleveland Browns
Former Defensive Coordinator, New York Giants

Carl Banks is a great role model for young people. He is honest, dedicated, considerate, and responsible. Football has been good to Carl and he wants to give something back to the game. This book, which does an excellent job of preparing beginning athletes to play the game, was inspired by that wish.

Carl is a very charitable man. He spends a lot of time with young people and is one of the first players on the Giants to offer help to rookies and other new players when they join the team. As a player, Carl possesses two qualities that great players always have: He is always in top condition and he's perfected the techniques of his position. By always giving 100 percent in practice and games, he continues to improve. A true professional, Carl always puts winning and teamwork above personal achievement and rewards. He has earned the admiration and respect of his teammates, coaches, and opponents and was a dominant force in the success of the Giants' defense during the eighties, including our 1986 championship season.

I have many memories of plays and deeds that Carl has done, but two stand above all others.

One incident I can vividly recall occurred in the 1986 NFC championship game against Washington. As usual, Carl was playing outside linebacker. The Redskins had fallen behind and were throwing on virtually every down. Just before halftime, Lawrence Taylor got hurt. Carl moved from his normal position to assume Lawrence's, and we put a substitute, Andy Headen, in Carl's place. Although he was playing a new position, Carl played one of the best games of his career.

We won the game, 17–0, which put us into the Super Bowl. Everybody in the locker room was ecstatic and jubilant. But Carl was so exhausted, he couldn't do anything but lie on the floor, spent from the effort he had put into the game. Though too tired to celebrate, he was just as happy as the rest of his teammates.

The other game took place in Atlanta in 1988. We were behind by ten points and there was some griping among the defense because we didn't think we were playing that well. From the middle of the second quarter on, Carl kept saying, "Just hang in there, play your position, keep playing hard, we're going to make the big play, you've got to believe in yourselves." He assured everyone we were going to get the job done.

But Carl was the one who made the big play. Actually, two big plays. His pressure on the quarterback led to Harry Carson's interception, which set up the tying touchdown. Minutes later, Carl intercepted another pass and returned it fifteen yards to give us a 23–16 victory. It was a perfect example of what his positive influence and dogged determination can do for the Giants in a game.

I am grateful for the opportunity to coach such an outstanding player and person. With this book, you will learn a lot about Carl, as well as how to condition yourself and prepare for a football season. Those are subjects that Carl Banks is exceptionally qualified to explain.

INTRODUCTION
TO THE PROGRAM

Whenever I think of what took place at Atlanta's Fulton County Stadium late in the afternoon of October 23, 1988, it will instantly bring a huge smile to my face and a warm feeling in my heart.

My team, the New York Giants, was losing to the Atlanta Falcons 16–9 with less than three minutes remaining in the fourth quarter. Our kicker, Paul McFadden, had just kicked a 45-yard field goal to reduce our deficit from 10 to 7 points. But with time ticking away and Atlanta in possession of the football, we were still in a difficult situation.

We had just used our third and final time-out with 2:54 left in the game. The Falcons faced a third-and-three from their own 32. If they had succeeded in getting a first down, they might have been able to hold the ball for the remainder of the game. Only the two-minute warning would delay the finality of a disheartening and unexpected defeat.

Atlanta quarterback Chris Miller dropped back to pass. After delaying for a second, I took off after Miller from the left side of the defensive line. Not one Falcon touched me. When Miller finally saw me, it was too late. I smashed into him and the ball went straight up into the air. When it came down, my teammate Harry Carson was waiting for it. He grabbed the ball and held on. Suddenly, it was our ball on the Atlanta 32.

Four plays later, Ottis Anderson scored from a yard out to tie the score at 16–16 with 1:57 remaining.

The Falcons took possession again, this time on their own 20. Hugh Millen was the new quarterback in place of Miller, who had suffered a pinched nerve in his elbow as a result of our collision. A false start penalty moved Atlanta back 5 yards. John Settle regained three of them on a run up the middle.

Now it was second-and-12 at the 18. I was lined up on the left side, close to the line. Millen took the snap and looked for a receiver

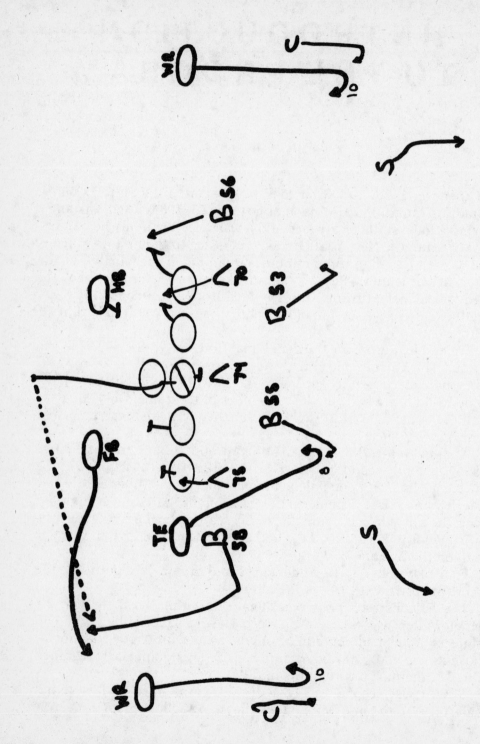

This play will always be one of the highlights of my football career, because it was the first touchdown I ever scored. On October 23, 1988, I intercepted a pass by Atlanta quarterback Hugh Millen and returned it 15 yards for the touchdown that gave the Giants a 23–16 victory. As this diagram shows, Millen was trying to complete a pass to running back John Settle when I stepped up, picked off the ball, and carried it to the end zone.

downfield, but found no one open. He then tried to complete a pass to Settle, who was flaring out to my side. I saw what was happening, stepped in front of Settle, and intercepted the ball.

Nothing but 15 yards of natural turf stood between the end zone and me. I took off, stumbled a bit near the goal line, but reached my destination untouched. My touchdown gave us the lead for good with 1:24 remaining. We won 23–16, in perhaps the most memorable comeback of the season.

That score was important for so many reasons. It gave us a victory in a game we seemed well on our way to losing just minutes before. The victory was our third in what would become a four-game winning streak. And it enabled us to remain tied for first place with the Washington Redskins.

On a personal level, I was able to enjoy my first touchdown. Ever. I had never before scored a touchdown in professional football. Nor did I score one in college at Michigan State, or at Beecher High School in Flint, Michigan. In fact, I had never known the thrill of carrying the ball over the goal line in junior high school or even in elementary school, when I played for the Daly Elementary School Tigers in the Men's Club League in Flint, Michigan.

Oh, but I almost did. That initial touchdown in Atlanta ignited the memory of the score I almost had back in the sixth grade. At the same time, it brought back a lot of wonderful recollections of playing youth football.

When I was in the sixth grade, we played the Zinc Mustangs for the championship of our league. I was a tight end. We used to run double reverses all the time, but I seldom got to keep the ball. Most of the time I was the handoff guy; I'd give the ball to another end or back who then ran the ball up the field.

We were losing the game in the fourth quarter and were backed up on our own 30, a full 70 yards from where we needed to be. Our coach, Rosey Haywood, called a fake double reverse and told me to keep it. In the championship game! I couldn't believe it.

I remembered the steps I had to make and how long the count was before I had to turn and get the ball from the running back. I got the ball and faked the handoff to Terry Russian, which fooled most of the defense. The Zinc players thought he had it, because they knew he was the one who usually got the ball.

But I had it. There I was streaking up the sideline. No one was even close to me. All I had to do was beat the free safety and I would have scored the touchdown. The safety's name was Duane Thomas.

This guy was very small, so there was no way he was going to prevent me from scoring.

But he did. I ran 69 yards and was just three feet short of the goal line when Duane Thomas flipped me in the air. I looked like a gymanstics star dismounting from the balance beam. When I finally landed, I was still on the 1-yard line. I did not score my first touchdown. I still don't know how little Duane Thomas did that.

All of the players and coaches from the league were there, because it was the title game. My parents were there. All of a sudden, the crowd was going crazy. It wasn't because of my great run, but the touchdown-saving tackle that Duane had made.

The worst part about the whole incident was that they held us at the 1-yard line. We didn't score and lost the game.

Playing for the Daly Elementary School Tigers began my love affair with the game. We were disciplined at practice, but I thought the entire experience was fun. We were taught right away that we had to be at practice on time and we had to learn all the plays. But those rules were fine with me, because I always wanted to get to practice and all the plays were fun to run. Everyone was involved in them.

That was very important. If you're going to play football, you have to enjoy it, but you also have to know how to play the game. That's why Coach Haywood was so great. He disciplined us, but he let us enjoy the game. He taught us very early the proper way to tackle, the correct way to execute plays, and how to avoid injuries.

This is my objective in this book. I strongly believe that my responsibility as a professional football player extends beyond the field of play. Throughout my career, I have tried to be a model example for children and adolescents, both athletically and by the way I handle myself off the field.

From my observations and discussions with youngsters, I know that kids need instruction and guidance if they are to enjoy youth and high school football.

With this book, you will learn about conditioning, about executing the fundamentals of the sport, and will receive advice in matters such as nutrition and refusing drugs.

Ever since I was a high school player I have been aware of the need to stay in proper conditioning during the off-season. It is even more important for me today and I think staying in good shape during the off-season should be a goal of yours.

If you arrive at pre-season training camp out of shape, you are inviting fatigue and injury. You won't be able to keep pace with your teammates who have worked hard during the off-season, and you will likely lose whatever opportunity you had to get a lot of playing time.

I never wanted that to happen to me, so I began to devise my own off-season conditioning program. Through the years I have added new segments to the program while deleting those I no longer considered effective. I now have a solid, cohesive, and challenging workout program that I adhere to every off-season. It enables me to build my stamina and endurance, increase my strength, and stretch my muscles to their maximum flexibility before I even hear a coach's whistle. It helps me get ahead of the game long before the games have started.

This is a comprehensive and complete program to get you in peak condition and prepare you for the football season. It can be applied to any sport that demands a great deal of aerobic movement. It helps you increase your strength. And it provides guidelines for healthy eating.

The program gets you into top condition steadily and gradually, which greatly reduces the risk of injury. It is a very safe plan, but at the same time it is thorough and demanding. You will work on a week-by-week and step-by-step schedule, with each week and every step designed to take you closer to your optimum condition.

If you want to get all you can out of this program, you have to get into condition to get into condition. You can't begin by running sprints and lifting heavy weights. That's a quick fix that simply won't work.

If you were a sprinter, your sole means of conditioning would not be a 100-yard dash. You would run much farther than 100 yards to build up your strength, endurance, and stamina, which will enable you to be much more successful when you do compete in a 100-yard race.

Before running sprints, you have to get yourself in condition. You don't want to traumatize your muscles or cause them to pull or strain by trying to do too much too soon. It's like learning to swim. You don't immediately jump into the deep end. First you have to learn how to stroke your arms and kick your feet in shallow water.

The same rules apply in conditioning yourself for the football season. You will get more out of the sprinting you will do in the latter half of the program if you condition yourself early. You have to set goals each week and stick to them.

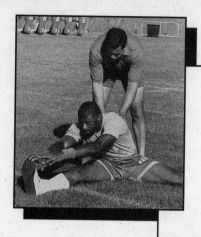

There isn't enough time to get in shape during the football season. You must arrive at pre-season practice in top condition.

If you are starting to work out after a long layoff, it's best to do some long-distance running—a mile or a mile and a half—to get your body accustomed to exercise. As the program progresses, you will increase your workout load.

The ultimate objective of this plan is to get into shape to play football. During the program, you will do different exercises, so you won't get tired or bored. Each exercise will address a different aspect of your conditioning. At the same time, they will all help you reach your primary goal.

Each day will begin with a crucial component of the program: stretching. It will prepare your muscles for the more demanding running and weight work while greatly reducing the risk of a tear or pull. Stretching also decreases your overall susceptibility to injury during the season by helping to prevent trauma to the muscles.

You will run long and intermediate distances, which will help develop your leg strength and endurance. The sprint work you do will benefit your cardiovascular recovery and accustom you to the high-speed situations you will experience during games and practices.

Another important aspect of the program is weight training, which is a supplement to the overall conditioning that is especially important to football players. As a football player, it is very important to have the muscle strength and conditioning, which running cannot create. The stronger you are, the better you perform. Increased strength also reduces your risk of injury. And if you are a strong person who is in condition, you will likely heal faster if you do sustain an injury.

A lot of the injuries suffered by football players are directly related to muscle strength. If you pull or bruise a muscle, the strength is automatically zapped from that area. The stronger you are, the less chance there is of that happening to you.

The nutritional recommendations tie in with the rest of the program. You have to eat healthful foods to get in peak condition. If you eat a lot of junk food, it's going to make your conditioning much more difficult. When you're eating a lot of fatty foods it is difficult to develop your muscles, because not enough nutrients get to the muscles. All your energy is spent burning off the junk in your system.

If you are striving to be a well-conditioned athlete or a football player, you cannot ignore even one component of my program. If you eat the right foods and you lift weights, you will become very strong. But if you don't do the prescribed running, you'll find yourself getting tired in a short period of time: the staying power so essential in sports will be missing.

Conversely, if you do all the required running exercises but rarely visit the weight room, then you won't be strong enough to play the game. You'll be knocked around a lot, because your body won't be able to withstand the pounding. You will suffer a lot more bumps and bruises and they will heal a lot slower.

The program takes 10 weeks to complete and will prepare you for training camp. That, in turn, will enable you to focus your attention during pre-season practices on your mental preparation, instead of worrying whether or not you are in condition to keep up physically. You should find out when your team begins its pre-season practice and start this program two and a half months prior to that date.

This program gives you a chance to gradually work your way into condition. That is the safest and most effective way to get into shape. It's not a crash course, which means its benefits will last a lot longer. It takes about 10 weeks to achieve total conditioning. At the completion of this program, you will be very close to peak condition.

My program can be undertaken by athletes in almost any sport. It isn't difficult and can be adapted and used by anyone. By following my plan, a youngster will improve his physical condition tremendously, even if he has never picked up a football.

This is the same program I use every year in preparation for the

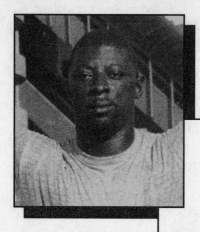

Make sure you are well rested for the start of pre-season practice.

grueling NFL season and it has grown out of the many exercises and techniques I have learned since I began playing. I have woven them together to form a cohesive system that, importantly, isn't very difficult and costs very little.

For anybody who plays it the way it should be played, football is a fun, competitive, and very physical game, but I wouldn't classify it as violent at any level or dangerous. Football is a game of controlled aggressions.

Before I began playing for Daly Elementary, I didn't believe I could have so much fun playing football. I was born in Chicago, where I was a fat kid who appeared headed for anything but athletic stardom. When I was very young I was lazy and had little motivation to play football.

But my family moved to Flint, Michigan, when I was eight and I became involved in sports, a part of my life I immediately began to love. Even as a kid I was concerned with conditioning. I ran everywhere and did push-ups, sit-ups, and sprints to keep myself in tip-top shape. At the same time, I was learning the correct way to play football.

All the hard work paid off for me. At Beecher High School in Flint, I was voted to All-State teams in football, basketball, and track (as a shot-putter). Truthfully, my favorite sport at Beecher was basketball. But I was neither tall enough nor good enough to make a career out of it.

So it was football I played at Michigan State, which is located a bit up the road from Flint, in East Lansing. In my senior year, I was named to four different all-America first-team rosters and was the team MVP. I was the Spartans' captain my junior and senior seasons, and when I graduated, my 287 tackles were the third-highest number in school history. I was the ninth player in the 87-year history of the Big 10 to earn All-Conference honors in three consecutive seasons. I am equally proud of the degree I earned in communications/public relations.

The New York Giants made me their first pick in the 1984 NFL draft, the third choice overall.

My early training and experience has played a major part in the success I now enjoy. The different disciplines it took for the Daly Tigers to run a play successfully have stayed with me through high school, college, and professional football.

When I arrived at my first professional training camp, I wasn't sure what to expect. But I worked extremely hard in my conditioning program during the off-season and I stayed late for extra practice when camp sessions ended. We had a lot of material to learn in a short period of time, but I was determined not to fall behind and I didn't.

In my rookie season, I played in every game and started four at strongside outside linebacker. The first time I started, I had ten solo tackles, two quarterback sacks, and a fumble recovery in a 19–7 victory over the Atlanta Falcons. That performance earned me the award as Sports Illustrated's Defensive Player of the Week. When the season ended, Pro Football Weekly, the Pro Football Writers Association, Football Digest, and United Press International all named me to their All-Rookie team.

The following year, 1985, I won the starting outside linebacker position and was playing well when a sprained knee knocked me out of action for four weeks. I returned in time to contribute to the last several games of the season and I made nine tackles in our two play-off games that season.

Like everyone else connected with and rooting for the Giants, the 1986 season will always be very special to me. Our overall record was 17–2 and I had the thrill of my football life when I started in Super Bowl XXI, where the Giants beat the Denver Broncos, 39–20. Individually, I led the team in total tackles with 120 during the regular season and 26 in our three-game post-season march to the championship.

Just as 1986 had been such a triumph for the Giants, 1987 turned into a huge disappointment. We lost our first two games, then missed four weeks because of a players' strike. During that time, a team of replacement players lost all three games it played. The Giants finished 6–9, including 6–6 in non-strike games, and missed the play-offs. We didn't even give ourselves a chance to defend our title.

Individually, I had a fine season. I again led the team in tackles with 113 and had a career-high nine quarterback sacks and my first career interception. My peers elected me to start for the NFC in the Pro Bowl in Honolulu and most major wire services and organizations selected me for their All-NFL teams. I was honored to be recognized for my play, but I would have traded every one of them for a chance to play in the Super Bowl again.

The next season, 1988, is one I'd like to forget. Because of a contract holdout, I missed all of training camp. I played with several nagging injuries throughout the season and my performance was far below what I had come to expect from myself. Worst of all, we lost the season finale to the New York Jets in the waning seconds, knocking us out of first place and the play-offs.

The Giants and I both made comebacks in 1989. The team was 12–4, the second-best record in the league, and won the NFC title.

I had my best season, with 97 total tackles and I set a team record with seven forced fumbles. We ran several defenses that enabled me to utilize my skills as an inside, as well as an outside, linebacker. It proved once again that you need to work on all your football skills, because you never know when you'll be called on to use them.

The hard work and success I had paid off in my selection as the NFC Most Valuable Player by the Washington Touchdown Club. Aside from winning the Super Bowl, that is the biggest honor of my career.

In many ways, my dreams have come true in the NFL. I have played on a Super Bowl champion team and lined up for the first play in the Pro Bowl. I am very proud of my success, but I don't dwell on it.

In the NFL, we play a grueling 16-game schedule. A pro athlete must get in shape before the season begins and maintain his strength and conditioning throughout the campaign. I recommend that you follow that same strategy.

There simply isn't enough time to get in shape during the season. So much needs to be done each week preparing and planning for the game. During the season, you must concentrate on your mental preparation: how you are going to play your opponent, what he is most likely to do in certain situations, etc. You cannot concentrate mentally if you're worried about whether you're in shape to play four quarters.

As a professional athlete, I realize that football is a year-round sport. The work I do during the off-season not only prepares me physically, but it sets my mental frame of mind for the coming season. The harder I work in the months when I'm not playing, the easier it is to maintain my concentration and a positive attitude during the season.

My off-season program consists of stretching, running, weight lifting, and drills designed specifically for football players. It's a basic yet effective program that will get you in shape. It is not the only program, but it has been an extremely effective one for me and for others. If your football coach or conditioning coach has a better plan, then you should listen to him until you've had a chance to figure out for yourself what gets you in the best condition.

My philosophy, and one I strongly recommend to you, is to always follow a coach's instructions. But a conditioning program designed by your coach might be very general, because it is designed to get the entire team in shape. Not all players on the team are the same. Many times, it takes an extra effort beyond what the coach is asking in order to be a better football player.

Getting in excellent physical condition takes more than running and lifting weights. You also need to adhere to a proper diet, drink the right fluids, and get plenty of rest. I have sought the help of a man I have tremendous faith in, Ronnie Barnes, to assist me with that portion of the program.

Barnes is the Giants' head trainer. An expert in nutrition and sports medicine, he has helped dozens of players with their nutritional needs, whether they are trying to gain or lose weight, or simply trying to maintain the weight they have. His ideas and beliefs carry a lot of force among the players in the Giants locker room.

Ronnie stresses the need to stay away from foods that are high in fat and believes in eating foods that have plenty of carbohydrates. He would much rather see athletes drinking water, fruit juice, and skim milk than carbonated sodas that have a high sugar content.

If you stick to the nutritional guidelines he outlines in the following chapter, you will have a significant advantage as you go through my workout program. You will be taking a huge step toward good physical conditioning.

To be in excellent physical condition is a great feeling. It changes my entire outlook on what I think I can accomplish, both on and off the field. Once you are in shape, everything else is relatively easy. You are functioning on all cylinders and can concentrate on the mental demands of your game.

Being in good condition has countless benefits away from the football field. When practice is over, you have the strength to do what you want to do or have to do. If you're out of shape and have had a rough practice, the only thing you want to do is sleep. You don't even want to eat, which would not make Ronnie Barnes—or me—very happy.

Good physical conditioning is a virtue with no negative side effects. If you do one thing for yourself, get your body in top condition. You will be happy you did.

PREPARING
FOR THE PROGRAM

The successful completion of my 10-week program is going to require a lot of hard work and determination. But before you stretch your hamstrings for the first time, or take that first run around the track, you're going to have to do some thoughtful preparation. If possible, find a partner to do the program with you. You can help each other with many of the exercises, and provide encouragement when the program becomes demanding.

Let's start with your clothes. You probably own several pairs of blue jeans that you love to wear during most of your waking hours, whether you're at school, the movies, or playing football. They might be in style and be very comfortable, but you are going to have to leave them home for the workout.

Jeans, or any other pair of pants that you would wear on any normal day, restrict your movement. They don't allow you to stretch fully, and stretching is a vital foundation of my program. It's impossible to do a butterfly stretch for your groin if you are wearing jeans. Either you're going to split your jeans, or, if you try to save your pants, you won't be able to get a full stretch. In addition, you won't be able to run properly in your everyday pants.

When you work out in this program, it is important that you wear loose clothing. Wear a pair of loose athletic shorts or sweatpants, depending on what the weather dictates.

On the upper half of your body, wear a loose-fitting T-shirt, tank top, or sweatshirt. Don't wear a tight shirt that restricts your movement in any way. Also, don't wear a rubber exercise top, because the excessive sweating it causes will likely result in your becoming dehydrated.

Make sure you wear a pair of white socks. It is always important to have a pair of socks on, at least while you are running. They give your ankles a little more stability. It's not a lot of stability, because

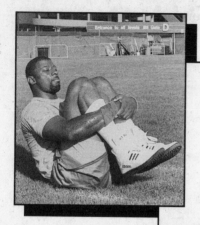

Wear workout clothes that are comfortable, including shorts or sweatpants, a loose-fitting T-shirt, white socks, and a good pair of running shoes.

you will be running in low-top running shoes, but it does give you some measure of support. Socks also help prevent blisters.

Get a good pair of running shoes. You are going to be doing a lot of running and exercising in the next 10 weeks. If you are trying to run in sneakers that are uncomfortable, it's going to make your task much more difficult and cause you a lot of pain. If your sneakers cause blisters, you will have to run in agony or take time off until they heal. That is time you may not be able to get back.

Your running shoes should give you adequate support while at the same time be comfortable enough to wear during long stretches of physical activity. Don't get very light shoes, like those that long-distance runners wear. They won't hold up when you start exerting yourself while sprinting the shorter distances later on in the program.

You must also pay close attention to and adhere to the dietary guidelines specified by Ronnie Barnes.

Ronnie has always stressed to the Giants players the importance of a proper, healthful diet. He has taught us how we put ourselves at a disadvantage if we don't eat the right foods.

You simply won't succeed in this program if you don't eat healthful meals. You may have an intense desire to do everything asked of you and to successfully complete the program as a prelude to your football season. You may be very motivated, but your body is going to stop if you don't give it enough of the proper fuel.

If you are trying to do the Carl Banks workout program without eating properly, you are simply not going to have the energy to complete the workouts. You will be too fatigued to reach your conditioning goals.

Start preparing yourself early. If you are subsisting on a diet that is heavy in fast-food hamburgers, french fries, doughnuts, ice cream, and sodas, begin eating better foods at least a week before you begin the program.

Ronnie has taught us that you don't eat today for today's workout. What you ate yesterday or the day before fuels your workout today and tomorrow.

So start now. And follow a few basic guidelines. Eat as many low-fat foods as you can. Fat is dead weight, it takes a long time to exit from your stomach, and it doesn't fuel exercise. Get your protein from poultry, fish, and lean meats instead of a fatty burger from the local fast-food chain.

Get as many carbohydrates as you can. Carbos give you the energy you need to keep your body functioning at an optimum level during workouts.

Where can you get your carbohydrates? From the same food sources we use in the Giants' diet. They include starchy vegetables, such as corn, beans, potatoes, and grains, such as rice and grits. More excellent sources of carbohydrates are fruits and fruit juices (not fruit drinks or fruit punch, which are little more than sugar water), breads, cereals, skim milk, or nonfat and low-fat dairy products. Oatmeal, pastas, and pizza are also good, but make sure you avoid the sausage and extra cheese on the pizza.

Start by eating a good breakfast. It's the meal that sets the tone for the rest of the day. If you don't eat a nourishing breakfast, you will be trying to catch up nutritionally for the rest of the day. Ronnie Barnes likes to say that if he could get players to do anything, it would be to make sure they all eat a healthful breakfast. He said that if you don't eat breakfast, your stomach will begin growling sometime during the morning. You will begin thinking about how hungry you are instead of the task at hand. Ronnie points out that in training camp, players who skip breakfast have a harder time paying attention to what is being taught in morning meetings, because they are daydreaming about eating lunch.

Eating a good breakfast is critical. I love doughnuts as much as anyone, but you can't eat doughnuts exclusively and expect to get through the program. This is not to say you have to cut them out of your diet. But try to cut down on those sugary, fatty pastry items

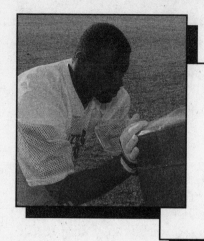

Eating healthy meals is essential for success in my program. Because fat is dead weight, eat as many low-fat foods as possible.

and stick to breads, rolls, bagels, or muffins. I've found an English muffin with jelly to be a tasty, healthful alternative to a doughnut.

Ronnie is also vocal in advocating a healthful lunch. He wants athletes to eat a carbohydrate-filled, high-energy lunch. You can do this by eating spaghetti, breads, vegetables, and potatoes. To get added fiber, he suggests a whole-grain bread.

Absolutely stay away from fried foods. They do nothing beneficial for you. They're high in fat and just not healthful. Eat fish at least twice a week. It is nutritionally sound and won't put fat on you. Eat turkey instead of ham-and-cheese. Use margarine instead of butter.

At dinnertime, poultry, fish, and other seafood are better than red meat, because they don't have as much fat. If possible, don't fry your poultry, and don't eat the skin. If you are going to eat steak, make sure it's nice and lean and not full of fat.

Complement the main dish with potatoes, rice, vegetables, and breads. Avoid added fat. Eat a lot of vegetables, like broccoli, spinach, and green beans. Have a salad with every meal, but cut back on fatty dressings, such as blue cheese.

Ronnie advocates drinking water, fruit juice, or skim milk instead of sugary, carbohydrate sodas. Those carbonated beverages make you feel fat and bloated. And when you drink soda, the sugar goes right to your stomach. Fluids follow it there instead of going to your arms and legs, where they could be used to help cool your body during exercise.

Barnes also believes you should reduce the amount of salt you consume. A good way to do that, he says, is to not add salt to your food.

Snacks and desserts can make a significant contribution to your nutrition. Stay away from the more expensive ice creams now on the market, because they are higher in fat content. As an alternative try soft-serve ice milks, low-fat frozen yogurt, or instant puddings that are made with skim milk.

If you want to eat between-meal snacks, try popcorn, preferably unsalted and unbuttered, fruit bar cookies, graham crackers, low-fat crackers, breads, and pretzels. Try to stay away from chips and nuts.

Without eating properly, you will probably find it very difficult to successfully complete the program. Ronnie points out that people who try strenuous exercise without adhering to a proper diet may feel stale and tired, and they may lack energy before and during workouts. You might even experience weakness, shakiness, difficulty in concentrating, extreme fatigue, all of which will certainly mean a shortened workout time.

For each day of the workout program, I have included a suggested menu. If you must deviate from the menus because of personal preference, please do so sensibly. The foods in the meals we have outlined are excellent for a young athlete working in a conditioning program. They will provide you with the fuel you will need for achieving your goals each workout day.

The timing of eating to exercising is very important. Ronnie and I

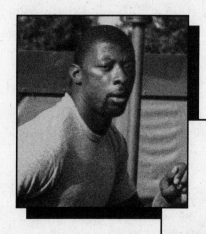

Eat a healthy breakfast every morning or you will be playing nutritional catch-up the rest of the day.

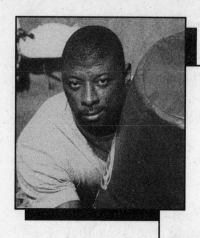

Maintain good dietary habits throughout the program.

Eat as many carbohydrates as you can.

Avoid beverages with caffeine, because they are dehydrating.

recommend that you wait at least 2 hours after a meal before working out. Give your body enough time to digest your food after you've had a big meal. Exercising too soon after eating can cause low blood sugar and result in shortened endurance—you might not be able to complete your workout. If you eat just before you work out, you'll be exerting yourself on a full stomach and when you try to run or lift weights, you'll be burping and risking nausea and vomiting.

Avoid getting into the habit of always eating when you're studying or watching TV. It's best to separate eating from other activities because over the long term you might get into the habit of eating every time you sit down, which makes it very difficult to control your weight.

Avoid extra caffeine, which is found in hot tea, canned iced teas, and colas. Caffeine is dehydrating and it is counterproductive to long-term weight control. It can also contribute to an increase in your blood pressure.

Learn now to stay away from alcohol. It has no place in a training athlete's diet. Alcohol increases your caloric intake while giving you nothing beneficial. It dehydrates you significantly. And, of course, it can badly impair your judgment. Do yourself a big favor and don't drink alcohol.

I like to get my running out of the way in the morning, especially in the summer, because then I'm not running in the heat. Heavy exercise in hot weather can be very damaging if you are not in condition or not prepared. Heat exhaustion is a common malady suffered by unprepared people who choose to exercise under mid-summer afternoon sunshine. The heat of summer afternoons can be very taxing and, besides, I get to work out under a broiling afternoon sun every day during training camp. I like to run when it's warm, but not too hot.

One of the most important issues for young athletes is fluid replacement. Dehydration can be life-threatening and must be avoided. In addition, a dehydrated athlete never performs as well as a hydrated athlete. If you are dehydrated, oxygen and other nutrients are unable to get to your muscles, because your blood volume is low. In addition, you won't be able to get rid of the heat that's produced during your workout, because you don't have enough blood to circulate to the working muscles and to the skin. Dehydration can cause lightheadedness or dizziness, and in hot weather that's when heat exhaustion can set in.

When you go to the track or field to work out, take a thermos or container of water or Gatorade. The latter is good, because it has sodium and a small amount of glucose, which helps speed the absorption of fluid. If you like, mix the water and Gatorade. During a game, the Giants drink half-strength Gatorade on the sideline.

During exercise, drink 8 ounces of water or watered-down Gatorade every 15 minutes. Don't wait until you're thirsty, because fluid replacement is an ongoing process. And dehydrated, fatigued

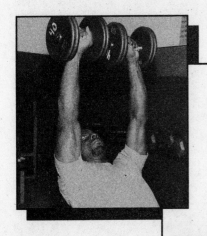

You can begin your workout at any convenient time of day, but always wait two hours after eating before you exercise.

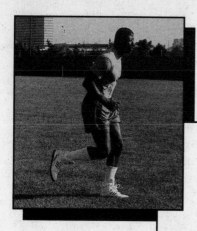

Always bring a fluid-replenishing beverage with you to the track and take a drink every fifteen minutes.

athletes get injured more frequently and take longer to heal than those who are properly hydrated.

Keep fluids handy at all times and drink them even if you don't feel thirsty. If you are sweating, you are losing fluid. You have to replace it, or you will fall behind in the program.

THE
PROGRAM

WEEK 1

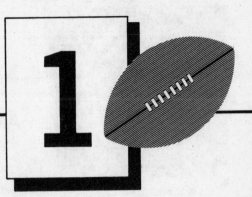

The first week should serve as a gauge. It is important to get a firm understanding of the shape you are in. Most of the work you will be doing this week involves stretching and running: flexibility is the key. In order to maximize your performance when the program becomes more difficult in the later weeks, it is essential to increase your flexibility now.

We will be working on speed and strength later on in the program. They are both important, of course. But you will fall short of your goals in those areas if you don't learn how to stretch properly now.

A word of caution: This is not the time to see how fast or far you can run or how much weight you can lift. In fact, weights are not even a part of this week's regimen. Remember, flexibility is the key this week.

The muscles you want to pay extra attention to in this early part of your training are the hamstrings, which are located in the back of the thighs; the quadriceps, the large muscles at the front of the thighs; the buttocks; and the calves. Those are the muscles you use to run. If they break down, you won't be able to run and your conditioning program will break down with them.

Throughout the program, your stretching will concentrate on these muscles. Toward the end of the regimen, your back muscles will become more important, because they can tighten up if you put too much strain on them.

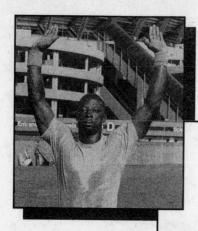

Always engage in a light warm-up activity before you begin stretching.

You don't want to shock your leg muscles and put too much of a strain on them too early. They need to be acclimated to the work you're going to be doing. It's vital to stretch all of them thoroughly and warm them up.

If you have tight leg muscles you have to take extra care, because sometimes it may be difficult to even stretch. For you to achieve peak condition, you have to reach your maximum flexibility.

MONDAY

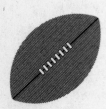

BREAKFAST: Let's begin the day, and our 10-week commitment, with a good, wholesome breakfast. Remember, you don't have to eat everything on the day's menu. But discipline yourself to avoid foods that aren't listed. Use the menus as a guide and stick to them.

Start with a glass of orange juice, apple juice, or other sugar-free juice. Eat a bowl of cold cereal that is not full of sugar, such as corn, bran or wheat flakes, shredded wheat, or Cheerios. Follow that up with pancakes and syrup or an English muffin and some cantaloupe. Eat honey, because it's a good natural sweetener.

▼

LUNCH: No more greasy hamburgers or peanut butter and jelly sandwiches for you. Try some baked chicken with mixed vegetables. If you have not completed your exercises for the day, eat a lighter meal, such as a chicken salad sandwich. Add to that a salad that includes lettuce, tomatoes, carrots, celery, and green peppers. If you have room for dessert, make it Jell-O, sherbet, or a piece of fruit.

▼

DINNER: Enjoy a big plate of spaghetti and meatballs, which is one of my favorite meals. Complement the main dish with bread and green beans. Don't drink soda pop. Instead, have some apple juice or water with your dinner. If you want dessert, try some sherbet or a banana. Stay away from cakes and ice creams that are high in sugar and fat content.

Be sure to drink extra fluids before you go to work out, particularly if it is a hot day.

A solid workout doesn't begin with running or stretching. You must first warm up, because stretching cold muscles puts you at a greater risk of pulling those muscles. A proper warm-up is needed, and stretching is not warming up.

Before you begin stretching, you should engage in a light warm-up activity. It must be something that enables you to break a light sweat, which is your indication that your body is warm enough to begin stretching. This can be a one- or two-lap jog around the track, which is what I usually do, or several minutes of running in place or doing jumping jacks. If you ride a bicycle to the track and are sweating when you arrive to begin your workout, then your trip to the track can serve as your warm-up. But always make it a point to warm your body up before stretching.

After your warm-up is completed, you should stretch for 30 to 40 minutes. This is not just to loosen you up for running, because the amount of running you will be doing this week isn't great. More important, it is to get your muscles ready for more work down the line. If you start out stretching properly today, and you keep doing it as I have described, it will become automatic to you as the program continues. Stretching will help you develop total flexibility, which should greatly reduce your chance of suffering a muscle injury once the football season begins.

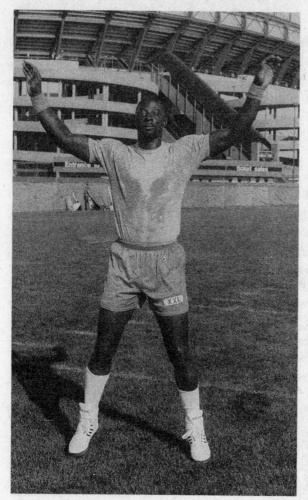
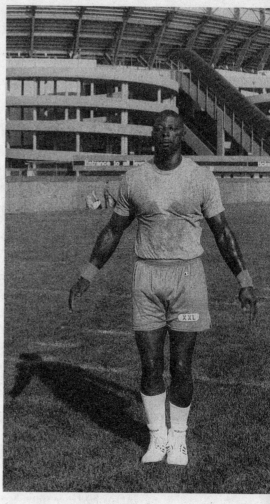

Jumping jacks are an
excellent way to warm
up before and after
stretching.

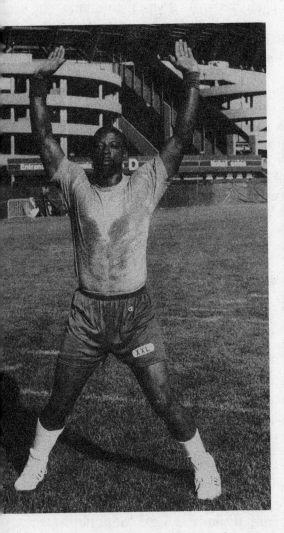

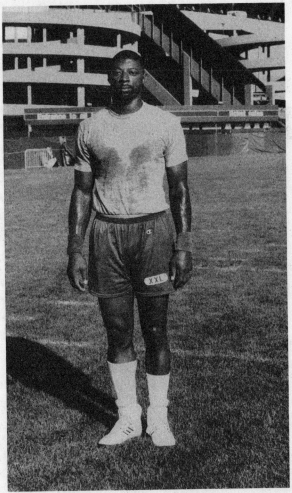

To prepare your body for the running you will be doing, it is important that you stretch every day. Without stretching, your muscles are in no shape to do any kind of running or exercise. If you put a lot of strain on these unstretched muscles, you can cause a pull or a tear. At the very least, you're going to experience muscle soreness. You won't avoid soreness by stretching, but you can greatly reduce it.

Your flexibility should improve each week. And you'll find that the more flexible you are, the more capable you are of accomplishing the things you need to accomplish. By being flexible, you can set more realistic goals for yourself in terms of improvement on a week-to-week basis.

Once I am warmed up I follow a regular, disciplined, and thorough stretching regimen that takes at least 30 minutes to complete. The exercises stretch the muscles in and near my legs, including the hamstrings, quadriceps, groin, buttock, and calf muscles, as well as the muscles in the upper body.

Every time I work out, I follow the same stretching routine, so I know each muscle is getting the proper attention before I begin more strenuous work.

Lower Body Stretching

I start with the *hamstrings* and I would suggest you do also.

You should pay specific attention to hamstrings because they are your most vital muscles when it comes to sprinting and are the key to your explosiveness in running. You have to make sure that your hamstrings are loose and warm. If you try to fire your hamstring and it's not ready, the muscle is going to pop. In the leg area, the hamstring is the muscle that is most susceptible to a pull or strain.

A major hamstring pull can take weeks or even months to heal. If you rupture a hamstring, it can take 6 months to heal and require extensive rehabilitation.

I pulled a hamstring in training camp my fourth year (1987) in the league. It was right after we had reported and we were doing our camp testing, which consisted of five 220-yard dashes. I ran three of them very well and I was feeling very good.

It was very hot and I took it for granted that the heat would help me stretch naturally. So I didn't stretch as long as I should have for five 220s. When I called on my muscles to respond for me when I was somewhat fatigued, they didn't. I pushed them too far and I

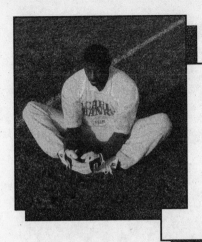

Stretching is just as important as running and weight lifting. Try to follow the same stretching routine every day, so you know you are not missing any muscles.

popped a hamstring. If I had taken more time to stretch and had gotten my muscles totally loose, then they would have been responding a lot longer during that workout. My hamstring wouldn't have quit on me after just three sprints.

The test called for five 220s and I shouldn't have had any problem, because I had done it many times. But when I tried to push myself to get a better time on the fourth one, the muscle pulled. Had I run them all at the same pace, I doubt that I would have pulled a muscle. But I was challenging myself and I didn't prepare myself for the challenge.

I missed four weeks of training camp because of that pulled hamstring. I had to sit out the first pre-season game at New England in 1987.

Before that day, I had always been very careful about getting in the proper amount of stretching. Since that one lapse, I've never taken warm weather for granted. Warm weather does help you get loose, because it's easier to break a sweat. But don't underestimate the work that you're going to do. Take the time to complete your stretching exercises. You can never stretch too much.

Begin by sitting on the ground, placing one leg straight in front of your body and bending the other leg behind you. This is called a *hurdler's stretch.* Go down and try to touch your head to your knee. You probably won't be able to get down all the way initially, but don't worry about it. Go down only until you feel a little pain. Get to

This is the *hurdler's stretch* position. When you bring your head down to your knee you will be stretching the hamstring muscle in the back of your thigh.

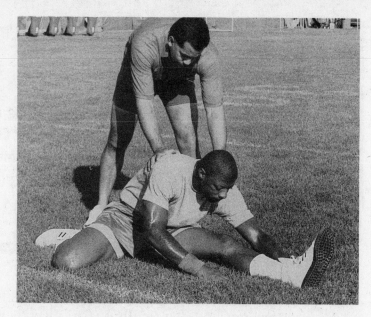

the point where you feel the hamstring stretching slightly and hold position there for 10 to 15 seconds.

You don't want to go until it really, really hurts, as that defeats the purpose of stretching by working the muscle too much. That in itself can cause a muscle strain.

After you do the exercise once, come up until you no longer feel the muscle stretching, then repeat the exercise. Do it 5 times. It's important not to bounce up and down when you're stretching, because you should stretch the muscle slowly and evenly. Reach your optimal stretching point and hold it there.

When you've finished stretching one leg, switch sides and stretch the other leg. Be as careful as you were the first time not to over-stretch, and discipline yourself to go down and stay down, without bobbing.

Another hamstring stretch is to lie on your back and raise one leg in the air. Grab that leg at the ankle or the thigh, whichever you feel more comfortable with, and try to touch your head to your knee. Get to a point where you feel your hamstring stretching and hold it for 5 seconds. Do that 10 times, then do the same thing with the other leg.

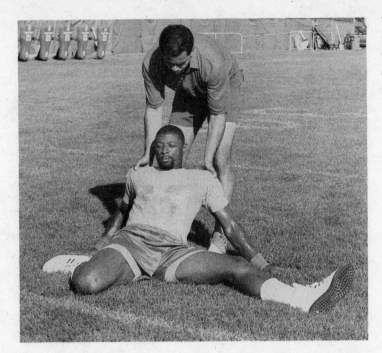

When you lean back in the *hurdler's stretch* you will be stretching the quadricep muscle in the front of your thigh.

Once you've completed this exercise, get back in your original hurdler's stretch. This time lean backward, not forward. Instead of your hamstrings, you will be stretching your quadriceps. Go down until you feel a pull similar to the one you felt in your hamstrings and hold it for 10 to 15 seconds. Repeat that 5 times with each leg.

After the quadriceps stretch, sit up with both legs spread in front of you. Spread them fairly wide, so the space between your feet is wider than the width of your shoulders. Go down on the right leg to a point where you can feel it stretching and hold for 10 to 15 seconds. I always alternate legs on this exercise, so I immediately do the same stretch on the left side. Follow this pattern until you have completed five stretches for each leg.

Since it is always a good idea to group similar stretches together, remain in the same position. This time, bring your head and chest down between your legs. In this position, you will be stretching the muscles of both legs at the same time. Hold for 10 to 15 seconds and repeat 5 times. Then lower your upper body while touching both feet at the same time. Hold for 10 to 15 seconds and repeat 5 times.

There are two ways to get an effective stretch on one leg when you are sitting on the ground with your legs apart. The first is to grab your foot and push your head down until you feel your hamstring stretching. The second is to bring your head down to your knee. I recommend you practice both methods.

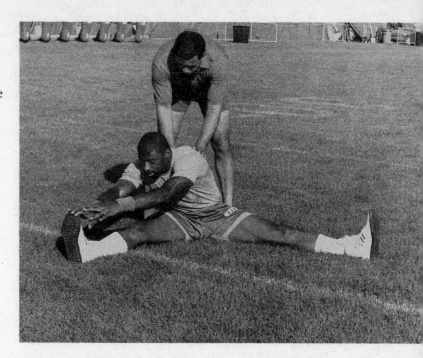

You can stretch both legs at the same time by keeping your legs apart and bringing your head down between your legs.

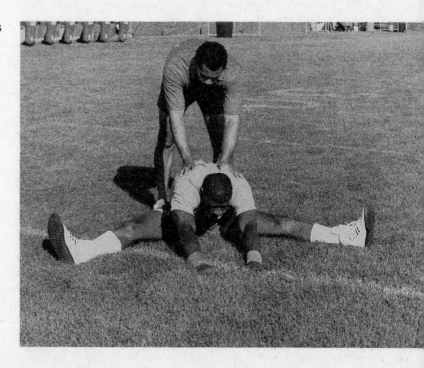

By now you should be feeling fairly warm. But your stretching routine is far from complete.

Remain seated and put your legs straight in front of you; they should be touching. Grab the toes of each foot and bend down until you feel that now familiar stretch in the hamstrings muscles. Hold that for 10 to 15 seconds and repeat 5 times.

My ultimate goal when doing this exercise is to put my head down far enough to touch my knees. You won't be able to do that right away, when you are out of shape. It takes a lot of time. You may not even get close when you're first starting out. But that doesn't mean you're not getting a good stretch. The entire first week you do this, go down only as far as the first time you tried it. This will help you guard against pulls. Your muscles will not yet be acclimated to the type of stretching exercises you're doing here, because you're not accustomed to stretching. It makes no sense to try to do too much too soon.

This exercise is a good one for measuring your progress. As time goes on, your head should get closer and closer to your knees. When

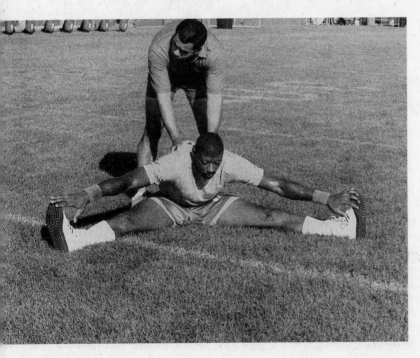

You can also stretch both legs at the same time by sitting with your legs apart and touching your hands to your feet.

To further stretch your hamstrings, keep your legs together, grab your toes, and bring your head down to your knees.

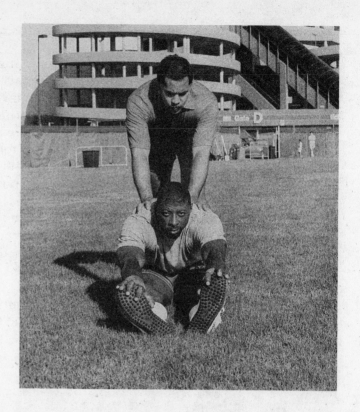

you can touch your head to your knees, you have achieved a milestone in this program.

When I am finished with that, I do the exercise that I call the *rocking chair.* I keep both my legs together and pull my knees up to my chest and hold them there so that it looks like I am tucked up into a ball. Once I am in that position, I rock back and forth on my back. This exercise loosens the back. Do it 10 times.

Once that is completed, I lie down with my legs and arms spread wide open. I look a little like a star. I then take one leg and try to touch it into the opposite palm while looking away. Don't look at the foot trying to touch your hand. That's why this exercise is called the *look-away.* It stretches the hamstrings as well as the back.

Early in the program, you almost certainly won't be able to get your foot into the opposite hand. And I suggest you don't try to actually put it in there until you feel comfortable or relaxed enough to do it. This should not be a painful exercise. None of the stretches

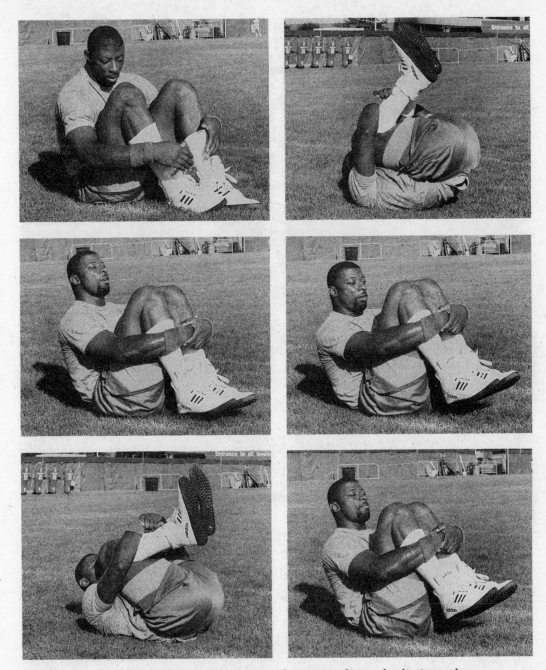

Your back needs to be stretched like any other part of your body. A good way to stretch your back is to sit on the ground, tuck yourself in a ball, and rock back and forth. We call this the *rocking chair*.

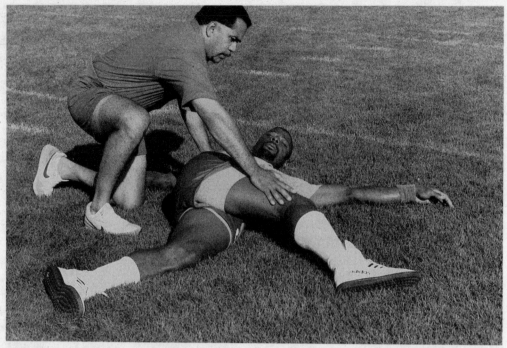

Stretch both your hamstrings and your back with this exercise, called the *look-away*. Bring your upper leg as close as you can to your outstretched arm.

should be painful. When you get to the point where you feel the muscle just starting to stretch, that's where you should hold it. Hold it for 10 to 15 seconds. I alternate legs, so as soon as I'm done with one side, I cross over and hold the other leg for 10 to 15 seconds. You will not have completed this exercise until you have stretched each side 5 times.

The groin is another very important area that needs to be stretched out. I can't emphasize that enough. This is where you can suffer a pulled muscle, and once you sustain a groin pull, you'll learn that they are very painful and very slow to heal. You always want to make sure you have that area stretched out.

While still on the ground, I sit up and put the bottoms of my feet together. I then grab my toes, point them up toward my chest, and push down on the inside of my thighs with my elbows. Hold it for 5 seconds. Repeat this 10 times. This is called a *butterfly stretch* and it

This exercise, called the *butterfly stretch*, enables you to stretch and tone an area of the groin that would be otherwise hard to reach.

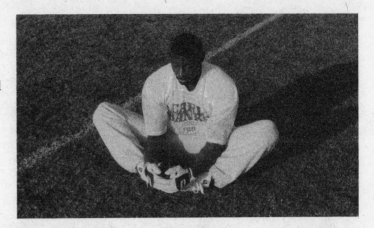

stretches the groin. The object of this part of the butterfly is to tone a part of the groin area that you normally couldn't reach. By pulling your toes up, you're stretching muscles high up in your groin.

I suffered a groin pull early in the 1988 season and it lingered for the rest of the season. It wasn't until after the season, when I was able to totally rest it for several weeks, that it healed completely. With most groin pulls, it will be four or five weeks before you can start any kind of activity.

After you have completed phase one of the butterfly stretch, you have more to do. Keep the bottoms of your feet together and push down on your thighs again. But this time, you're not pulling your

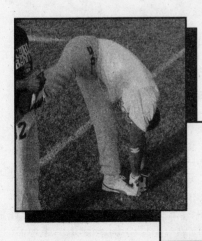

You are at greater risk of pulling a muscle if you don't stretch thoroughly, even late in the program.

You can reach muscles further down in your groin by placing the bottoms of your feet together and then pushing down.

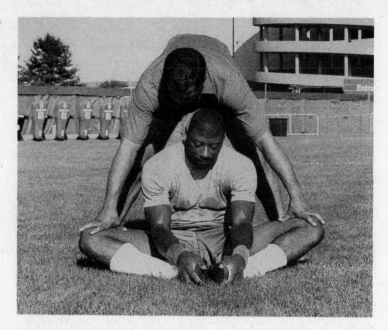

toes up toward your chest. You are simply pushing down. Because you're not pulling your toes up, you are stretching muscles a little further down in the groin area.

If you are working out on your own and you don't feel as though you have stretched your leg muscles enough, repeat the exercises I have just detailed.

If you are working out with someone else—and it is much easier to go through the workout program with a partner or two—there are other stretches you can do.

The first you should do is this: Stand up facing your partner and put one of your legs in your partner's hands; he holds it about waist high. In essence, you repeat your hurdler's stretch. As he holds your leg, you bend down toward that leg and try to put your head on your knee. Do that 5 times and hold for 5 seconds.

Again, it's not important to try and get your head touching your knee the first few weeks you're doing it.

If you have no partner, you can duplicate this stretch by putting your leg on a step or fence. But I wouldn't recommend that. You may get a fence that's too high and you won't be able to get down properly.

By working with a partner, you can increase the number of exercises you do. This one will enable you to further stretch your hamstrings.

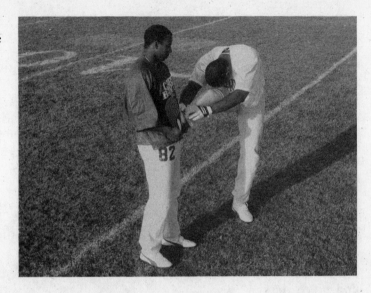

Once you have done that part of the exercise, and your partner is continuing to hold your leg, you should go down on the leg you have planted on the ground while keeping it straight. Try to touch your head to that knee. Repeat 5 times, holding for 5 seconds.

When you have finished putting your head down to each knee, switch legs and do the same stretching on the other side.

Don't squander stretching opportunities on the practice field. After you have stretched the leg that your partner is holding, put your head down and stretch the other leg.

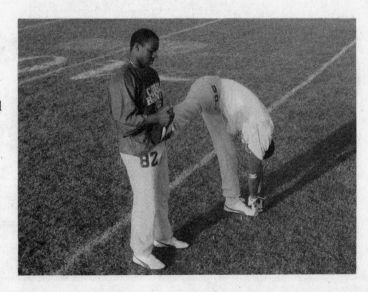

Upper Body Stretching

After you have completed stretching your lower body, then you need to loosen up your upper body. It is just as important for the upper body to be loose and stretched out before you begin working out on the lower body.

The first thing I do is stand straight up and make big arcs with my arms by rotating them in the air. I do alternating sets of 10 forward and 10 backward until I have done 40 each way.

Upper body stretching is very important. A good way to begin is to put your arms up and out to your sides and rotate them in large circles.

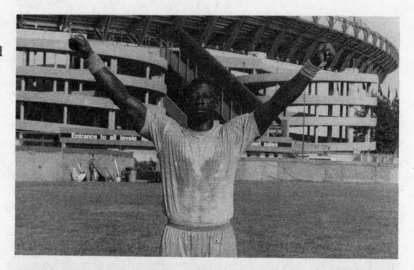

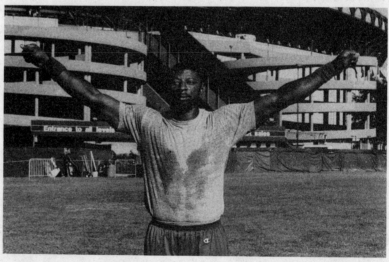

When that is complete, I hold my arms out to the side, put my feet together and twist, going from side to side. Don't bend your waist. Turn as if your feet are anchored to the ground, but you are trying to see what's behind you. This also helps loosen up the back. I do that a total of 40 times in alternating sets of 20.

After that exercise, I continue to keep my feet together. Then I put both arms over my head and stretch, as if I'm trying to pull a cloud down from the sky. Keep reaching and hold it for 5 to 10 seconds. I always do it 20 times, sometimes making a brief stop after 10.

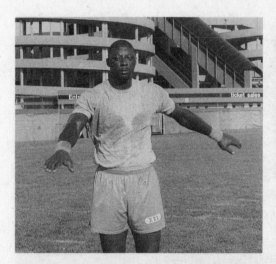
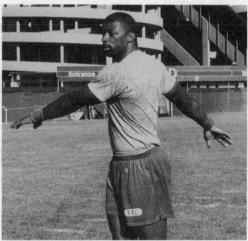
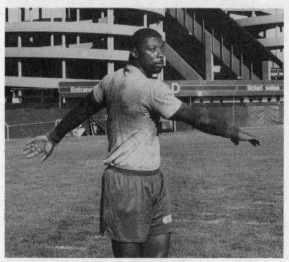

You can stretch the back and hip muscles by keeping your arms outstretched and moving your hips from side to side.

Once that is completed, I put my palms together and again reach upward. I do that 10 times. The palms-together reach stretches the shoulder muscles.

If you have a partner, there's another good shoulder stretch you can do. Put your arms behind you with your thumbs down, pointing toward the ground. Have your partner grab both your arms by the wrists and lightly try to push the palms of your hands together. Take extra care when doing this exercise. You have to be cautious that your partner doesn't try to just jam your arms together. He should lightly apply pressure or he could pull your shoulder out of its socket.

Midway through the program, you will probably start to feel that you are well stretched and don't need to spend 30 minutes stretching each day. That is wrongful thinking, and skipping your stretching routine would be a big mistake. You will never arrive at the track or football field with your muscles already stretched, because the muscles in your body don't stretch until you stretch them. You can't wake up, eat breakfast, wait for 2 hours, then go to the track and expect your muscles to be prepared for a workout. That's why it's so important to do these exercises every day. If you skip your daily stretching, you may very well pull or strain a muscle, and that could set you back for weeks.

If you feel your muscles are pretty well stretched, it may not be

A good way to stretch your shoulders is to have your partner hold your arms behind your back as you lightly try to push your palms together.

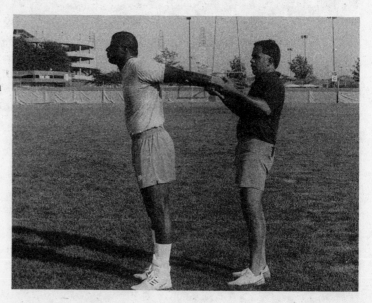

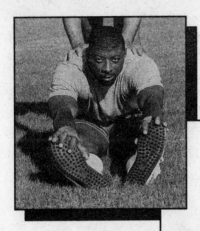

Don't cut short your stretching time, even at the end of the program.

necessary to do as many repetitions. But you have to do all the stretches, because they are what determine how loose you are. If you take for granted that your groin is loose, and you skip that exercise, that's probably the muscle you're going to pull. If you're doing the exercises, and you feel loose going through each one, then you can keep going on to the next one. You don't have to do as many repetitions.

I feel strongly, however, that there should be a certain amount of repetitions regardless of how loose you feel. I don't think you should ever do fewer than 10 repetitions of any stretching exercise. Some days I get to the track and I feel as loose and as flexible as a rubber man. But I still make sure I do at least 10 repetitions of each exercise. I often do 12, because I don't want to take anything for granted.

Remember: Reduce the number of stretching repetitions you do only after you have been stretching for several weeks and only if you genuinely feel that you are well stretched. Otherwise, don't even think about it.

After you have finished your stretching, it is a good idea to do about 15 *jumping jacks.* Stand straight with your legs together and your arms at your side. Jump up and kick your legs out while clapping your hands above your head. Do this 15 times without stopping. This gets your heart rate going and recaptures some of the body heat you may have lost during stretching, when you are relatively inactive.

Now you are ready for running. But that does not mean your stretching is finished for the day. Your muscles will tighten up after you run. So after you've completed your running or any other type of exercise, it's important to repeat the stretching process. This eases the pain that you will experience tonight. If you stretch before and after your exercises today, then tomorrow should not be so tough.

Don't stretch immediately after you have completed your running. Just as you warmed up before stretching the first time, now you need to warm down before you stretch again. To do this, walk a lap or two before you do post-exercise stretching. I always do my late stretching in the same sequence in which I did my stretching earlier.

One final word on stretching: I believe very strongly that it is just as vital as running and weight lifting. Stretching allows you to enhance your performance in all the other physical disciplines.

Stretching does not have to be limited to before and after your running exercises at the track or lifting exercises in the gym. When you have a few minutes at home, sit on the floor and stretch. There's no such thing as too much stretching. To get the most out of your exercises, you must have your muscles prepared. It's just like taking a test in school. You wouldn't do well in a test if you didn't prepare the night before taking it. On the athletic field, you can't do your best unless you are stretching. It is your preparation before the big test.

When you have finished stretching, take a drink. Try to take a thermos or jug filled with water or Gatorade to your workout. As I noted earlier, Ronnie Barnes believes fluid replacement is extremely important, particularly for young football players. Youth and high school football players are used to being active, but not in football pads in hot weather. That is a combination that could cause you to perspire more than you are accustomed to.

When you perspire, you lose bodily fluids. If you lose too much fluid, you can become dehydrated, which can become a life-threatening condition.

The way to avoid dehydration is by replacing the fluids you lose when you perspire. During your workout, drink about 8 ounces of fluid every 15 minutes. Make sure it is water or a fluid-replacement beverage such as Gatorade. Ronnie prefers pure water. I have tried

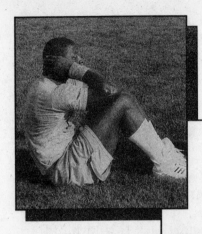

both and don't really have a preference. The important thing is that you have a fluid-replacement beverage available to you.

Don't drink carbonated beverages or iced tea. Carbonated drinks will fill you up and make you feel as if you would rather lie down than continue your workout. Iced tea has too much caffeine, which eliminates it as a good fluid-replacement beverage. And please don't drink alcohol in any form. Alcohol is dehydrating. If you try to hydrate by drinking an alcoholic beverage, you are defeating the purpose of drinking the fluid.

One of the ways you can avoid becoming dehydrated over time is to weigh yourself before and after every workout. If you find that you have lost weight after working out, you should replace each pound of weight that you lose with one pint of water. That's two 8-ounce cups of water or a fluid-replacement beverage like Gatorade. If you are 165 pounds before your workout and then weigh 162 following your workout, you should drink 3 pints of fluid. Once you get those in, keep drinking juices, water, or Gatorade throughout the evening.

Now that you have recharged yourself with a drink, it is time to take the program's initial test. In my program, you will be doing a lot of running.

Sports is running and running is the cornerstone of my workouts. You cannot succeed in football if you can't run. Long-distance running gives you the stamina and endurance you need when games reach the fourth quarter and the season grows long. Running shorter distances prepares you for the constant stopping and starting a football player does during a game.

Anyone who wants to get in top physical condition can take a big step simply by running. My program combines speed and distance work, which helps give me both explosiveness and staying power, two assets essential in football.

This week, you won't be doing running that is very strenuous. You don't want your muscles firing too fast or too rapidly, because your body is not in shape to accommodate that kind of demand.

You can set yourself back by running a 110-yard sprint if your muscles aren't used to it. You have to start slowly and build up gradually. I call this getting in shape to get in shape. You will slowly and gradually build up endurance and stamina. At the same time, you will be getting your muscles accustomed to running.

The explosiveness and stamina I gain during these off-season workouts helps me every time I put on my uniform. It really comes into play when we face the Philadelphia Eagles, which is a team with a large number of offensive weapons. The Eagles have Randall Cunningham, Keith Byars, Anthony Toney, Keith Jackson, Cris Carter, and Mike Quick. It takes speed and quickness to cover and tackle them, once I see where the ball is going. Everyone is strong at the beginning of a game. But I have to be able to get to them just as quickly late in the fourth period as I did early in the first.

That's where running comes in. Your running should be done on a track. It will help alleviate back problems and shin splints, two ailments you are more likely to suffer from if you run in the street. You also run a greater risk of stepping in a pothole or up on a curb and twisting your ankle if you do your running in the street. That's what happened to Tim Teufel of the New York Mets, who was jogging in the streets of Chicago when he turned an ankle early in the 1989 season. The injury forced him to go on the disabled list.

A track is a good place to run because you can measure distances, which will either be marked off or easy to gauge accurately if you know the size of the track.

Remember, you are not ready to run until you have completed your stretching.

No matter what kind of running you're going to do, it's a good idea to jog a half-mile to get your muscles used to running.

Between your half-mile jog and the beginning of your more stren-

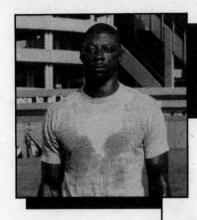

Do your running on a track, not in the street.

uous work, you should stretch for another 3 to 5 minutes to prevent you from completely cooling down.

If you are age twelve or younger, a half-mile may be all you need. If you wish to do more, walk a lap after your half-mile jog, then do ten 60-yard wind sprints. When you are done, jog a lap at a very slow pace to cool down. Once you complete your cool down lap, stretch as long as you did at the beginning of the workout.

For the older group, if you're just starting out with a running program, it's good to build some stamina and endurance.

Always rest enough between runs to catch your breath and gather your strength so you can do your next drill properly. This doesn't mean sitting down and admiring the sky. If you take a seat, your muscles are going to tighten up. The thing to do is walk a lap or walk the distance you have been running. If, for example, you are running 330 yards, take a 330-yard walk between and after your run.

When you run longer distances, your muscles become used to a longer stride. Shorter sprints are more explosive and the muscles stretch differently and have to react faster. For that reason, if you come right off a distance run and immediately try to sprint, you risk putting too much of a strain on your muscles.

It's very dangerous to go from a longer distance to a shorter distance without first stretching. Such stretching prepares you physically and mentally for the work you are about to do. It acclimates your muscles to the new type of exercises you are about to start. It's like running a 440, then coming back and running a 50-

yard dash. Mentally you have to prepare for it and, physically, the muscles have to be ready for it.

If you fail to stretch, you risk straining a muscle. Your muscles will be tired after a longer-distance run. You have to let them cool down, then stretch them to prepare for a shorter distance.

You should feel some muscle soreness at the end of the first few days of running and at the completion of your initial weeks of the workout, especially if you haven't worked out for a while. Your weekends will be your rest periods. If you feel a great deal of soreness, go out on one of the days over the weekend and do some light jogging. If you have access to a whirlpool or a jacuzzi, it's wise to use it as often as you can, especially when you're just starting out. If you don't, take a warm bath with Epsom salts.

Always be aware of your limitations. Don't try to do too much too soon. Mentally, you can become very discouraged, because you're not achieving what you set out to do. If your goals are too high and your body is not prepared to meet them, you will become exasperated and frustrated.

Physically, if your body is not ready to do what you are demanding it do, then your components are going to break down. It's like trying to drive your car a long distance on three good tires and one bad tire. The one bad tire is going to blow. If you try to do too much too fast, something is going to blow on your body. It might be a pulled or strained muscle, a sore tendon, or painful joints. It will set back your conditioning, because you will be spending more time trying to heal your injuries than on getting in shape.

If you feel you need to rest, take a break. But keep in mind that you are trying to get in condition and tired doesn't necessarily mean fatigued. You have to be the judge of how you feel. Don't take the easy way out by, for example, skipping exercises or taking too much time between exercises. If you know you can do more than what's prescribed in this book, then do it. If you're not getting tired from doing this program, you are not doing it hard enough. It's designed to get you tired but not flat-out fatigued.

The Running Program

My running program is divided into *four phases*. All of them prepare you for the type of running you have to do on the football field, which is repeated short bursts of speed.

The *first phase* is distance running. You may wonder why you have to bother with distance running if your goal is to be a football player. It may seem to you that you should be sprinting. But if you skip distance running and go right to sprinting, you'll have the same fleeting success that the hare had in his famous race against the tortoise. You'll start off fast, but you won't have the endurance to be a strong finisher.

Speed will come later on in the program. First you must build some stamina and endurance. Some people have it naturally. They were born with it and hardly have to work to maintain it. But it does require some tune-up.

You have to develop stamina and endurance by running distances of a mile, a mile and a half, and 2 miles. It's not necessary to exceed 2 miles; we're not training for the Olympics here. Also, we don't want our bodies to become so stretched out and limber from running distances that it would be difficult to run sprints later on. In the workout program, I will start you off on the path to peak condition with distance running.

Distance running develops your body so you will be able to exercise for longer periods of time. Without working your body into shape with distance running, you may feel strong for the first three quarters of a football game, but you could well feel fatigued for the final 15 minutes.

The *second phase* of my running program involves intermediate or middle distance work. This includes a 440-yard run and the half-mile. They are designed to further build up your endurance and your leg strength, as well as your overall conditioning, which will enable you to keep playing at top speed for a longer period of time. The middle distances help refine what the long-distance running has started.

The intermediates are not long-distance runs, nor are they sprints. You are developing your endurance while running faster than you would over a 2-mile distance, but not as fast as if you were running a 100-yard sprint. This is what I consider strong running. You often hear it said that so-and-so is a "strong runner." That is what the intermediate running does for you. It gives you strength in your running. You have to work harder, but not as hard as you will when you start sprinting.

Phase three includes sprint work with a touch of intermediate running. In this group are 220- and 330-yard runs. You are still building endurance, but you're picking up the pace a little more with the 220s.

Sit-ups are an important part of my program. Keep your legs anchored and when you come up, make certain you feel your stomach muscles working. If you don't, you are not doing the sit-ups properly.

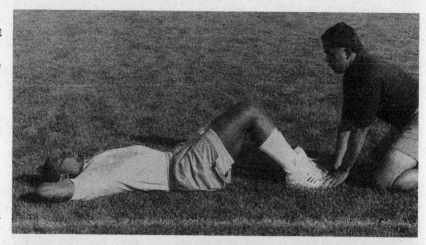

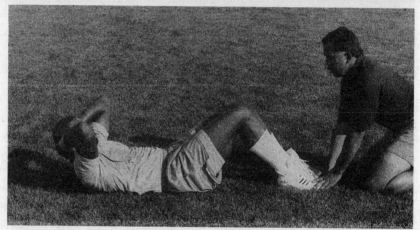

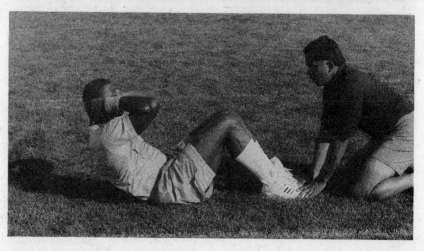

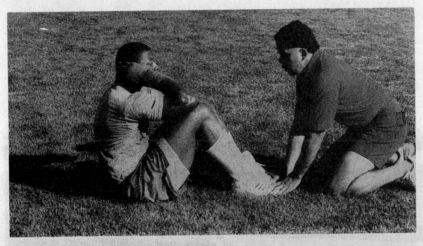

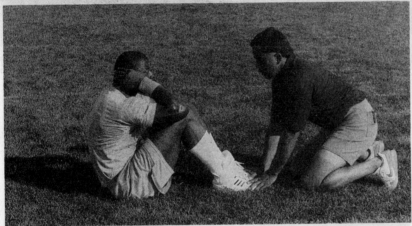

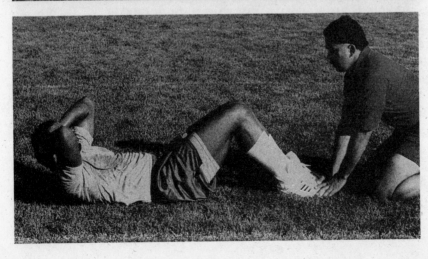

Keep in mind when you are in the program that as you go down in distance, you should be picking up the speed. You shouldn't run a 220 at the same pace you would run a 440. You should be gradually picking up speed and working a little harder to get the maximum benefit from your running.

The 220 is considered a sprint, but it is longer than a sprint. When you run it, you are conditioning yourself for explosion for a greater period of time. It's a longer run than you would need on the football field, but it conditions the muscles to develop endurance.

The *final phase* of my running program includes the shorter sprints. These are sprints of distances of 110 yards and less. When you get to this part of the program, you are running distances that are directly related to what you will be doing on the football field. These are the quick bursts with maximum explosion that you will need countless times during a football game.

When you get to this phase you really have to give it your all, because you are simulating how you are going to be running on the field. You can't allow yourself to jog a 110- or 60-yard dash. Whether you play offense or defense, that's not going to get you anywhere near what you need to be on the football field.

The shortest sprint I run is 20 yards. It helps me quickly get from Point A to Point B on the football field. It's a short sprint that requires the quick explosion that I need all the time as a linebacker chasing a ballcarrier from one side of the field to the other. The 20-yard sprint closely simulates what you do dozens of times during a football game.

The 60-yard dash helps prepare me to pursue the ball for distances greater than 20 yards. If a running back takes off through a hole, I have to pursue him. It can require running very hard for a longer time than I am accustomed to. Sometimes I don't have a direct line from Point A to Point B, but I have to get in position to chase the ballcarrier. A 60-yard dash prepares me perfectly for this.

The 110-yard dash improves my endurance for the two shorter sprints. I seldom run close to that distance in a game. But a 110 allows me to run for a longer period of time on a football field. It helps give me the strength to run faster longer.

You will often need that endurance during a game, especially if you are a running back. During a play, a back may run only 20 yards forward, but he may cut back and forth in several different directions to get there. That can add up to the equivalent of running

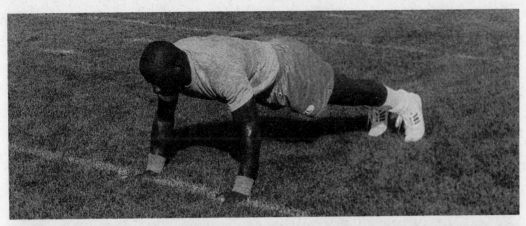

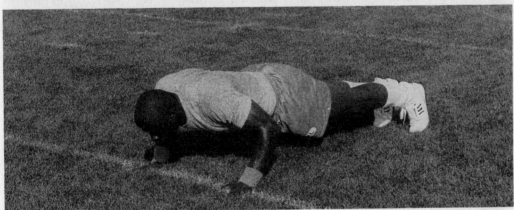

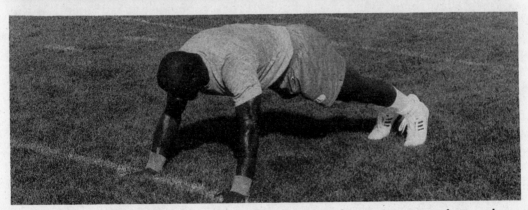

It is important to maintain discipline when doing push-ups. Keep your legs and back straight and bring your chest all the way down to the ground. When you go up, go far enough to straighten your arms.

forward 40, 50, or 60 yards. Not everything on a football field is run in a straight line.

Running is hard and can be very tedious. It requires tremendous discipline. To get the maximum effect out of it you have to stick to a schedule, such as the one I've laid out in my program. That can be difficult sometimes when your muscles are sore and you want to take a day off. If you do that you put yourself behind and set yourself up for suffering more pain and anguish the next time you do run.

I enjoy being in shape. I don't really enjoy running, especially when it gets tough in the middle of the program. But the benefits are very, very positive if you stick to it.

On this opening day of your pre-season workout, run 2 miles. Time yourself and record your time. Today's run doesn't have to be your top speed, but don't turn it into a walk, either.

After you've run the 2 miles, walk a lap to warm down. Then stretch for another 30 to 40 minutes.

When you have finished that round of stretching, do 25 sit-ups. You can keep your legs straight out in front of you or bend them at the knees. Choose the position that allows you to benefit most from the exercise. Sit-ups are designed to strengthen your stomach area, so if you think one position better serves that purpose, use that.

Finish the day with 25 disciplined push-ups. Make sure to touch your chest to the ground and fully extend your arms when you lift yourself up. Don't cut corners by going half-way down or half-way up. Keep your back and legs stiff and go all the way up and all the way down. Don't shortchange yourself because it is the end of the day.

TUESDAY

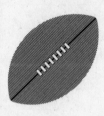

BREAKFAST: Start with a glass of orange juice. Continue with half a grapefruit, some French toast with syrup and, if that doesn't fill you up, a fruit Danish.

▼

LUNCH: Beef noodle soup with crackers, followed by baked macaroni and cheese. If you prefer to have a soup-and-sandwich combination, eat a roast turkey sandwich on whole wheat bread. Don't forget to include a salad. Drink water, fruit juice, or low-fat milk with your meal.

▼

DINNER: Have another salad here. For your main course tonight, try a Cornish hen with stuffing, green beans, corn, and dinner rolls (without butter). Stay away from sodas and drink fluid-replacement beverages with your meal. A banana or dish of peaches will make a nice dessert.

Throughout the day, drink enough fluids. Remember to have fluids with you while working out.

Warm up.

Stretch for one hour, paying particular attention to the hamstrings. Unless you've followed a conditioning regimen year-round, you are probably out of shape and the first muscles that will likely cause you problems are the hamstrings, because you will be using them so often. You want to get them flexible, so they will accommodate your body's movement and the type of running you will be required to do.

If you have tight hamstrings, you won't be able to accomplish very much: your muscles will tire faster and when they're tired, they stretch. A rubber band that's stretched too far pops. Your muscles can pop, too, which can sideline you for a long time.

So please stretch thoroughly and carefully.

WEDNESDAY

BREAKFAST: Kick-off with orange or grapefruit juice, then have some honeydew melon. We'll follow that with a couple of scrambled eggs and some potatoes or grits. Have a bowl of hot cereal such as oatmeal, cream of rice, or cream of wheat. Include honey somewhere in your meal, such as on a piece of toast.

▼

LUNCH: We'll stick to our healthful diet this afternoon with a turkey club sandwich and some egg noodles. Have to get those carbohydrates! Don't leave the table without eating a mixed green salad. Stick to the beverages that will help you when you work out.

▼

DINNER: I wasn't kidding about the carbohydrates. This evening we'll have both manicotti and rice, plus some bread or rolls. Complete the meal with some carrots. Tonight, we'll have a dessert treat with some ice cream, though I recommend you stay away from the hot fudge. If you want to maintain your discipline, eat an apple instead.

Don't forget to weigh yourself before working out. Replace fluids as needed.

Warm up.

Stretch for 30 to 40 minutes. If you don't feel that your muscles are properly loosened, take another few minutes. Don't ever take a shortcut through your stretching regimen, because it will come back to haunt you later on.

Jog three half-miles in the following manner: Jog a half-mile, walk a lap, jog a half-mile, then repeat once more. Time your half-mile runs and record the times.

Warm down.

Stretch for 30 to 40 minutes.

End the workout day as we did on Monday, with 25 sit-ups and 25 push-ups. If you are unaccustomed to doing sit-ups, your stomach may be a little sore from Monday's set. This is natural. If you can't do the full complement of 25 sit-ups, try to do as many as you can.

THURSDAY

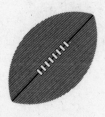

BREAKFAST: Start the day with a glass of your favorite juice. Continue with a cantaloupe or fruit cocktail, waffles with syrup or honey and, if that doesn't fill you up, a fruit Danish. Drink skim or low-fat milk with breakfast, if you like.

▼

LUNCH: Today we'll have soup and a sandwich, a quick and healthful meal. Have vegetable soup with crackers, plus a roast turkey or tuna fish sandwich on whole wheat bread. Don't forget to include a salad with your meal. Drink water, juice, or low-fat milk.

▼

DINNER: Tonight, try some baked filet of sole or flounder, with peas and/or lima beans and corn, plus rice. Make sure to have dinner rolls. Eat a salad if you like. Drink water, fruit juice, or low-fat milk. Eat an apple or peach for dessert.

Warm up.

Stretch for 30 to 40 minutes. If you have been keeping yourself in relatively good shape, then you may not have to stretch this long on the weekends. Only you can judge fairly and accurately what kind of shape you're in.

If you have been very inactive in the weeks and months prior to beginning this program, then you should stretch for an hour. It's going to take your muscles longer to get in condition than those of someone who's been working out regularly.

At this point, I think stretching is more important than running.

Jog at least a half-mile to a mile to loosen up. If you feel up to it, go a little further. But don't overdue it. This is just the first week and you don't want to do too much too soon. The focus now is getting your body into condition to get into condition.

Don't try to loosen up or speed up the conditioning process by doing wind sprints. At this point in the program, I think it's very unwise to try sprinting.

FRIDAY

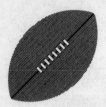

BREAKFAST: Start your day with a glass of apple juice and have half a grapefruit or half a pear. Continue with a healthful bowl of cold cereal, such as oat bran, wheat flakes, or puffed rice. Avoid pre-sugared cereals. Finish up with French toast, grits, and/or toast and honey. The Giants' trainer recommends honey.

▼

LUNCH: Open up with a bowl of chicken soup with crackers. We want to make sure you have the energy for the week's final workout, so have a plate of spaghetti or fettuccine with plain tomato or red clam sauce. If you think that's too much for you, substitute a turkey sandwich on whole wheat bread for the pasta. Include some carrots with your meal and make sure you eat a mixed green salad. Drink healthful beverages.

▼

DINNER: Treat yourself tonight with a sirloin steak, but make sure it is lean. Trim all the fat away. Include with your meal a baked potato and mushrooms, broccoli or boiled zucchini, and dinner rolls. Stick to water, juice, or low-fat milk. For dessert, eat a plum or an apple.

Weigh yourself before working out.

Warm up.

Stretch for 30 to 40 minutes. If you are feeling a twinge in your hamstrings, or one or two muscles are extremely sore, it means you are stretching too hard. If you feel a twinge, don't go down as far as you did earlier in the week. Go down enough so you feel them stretching, but not straining.

When you have finished your stretching, run 2 miles. Try to go a little harder than you did on Monday. Walk a lap to warm down.

Replenish fluids regularly.

Finish the day with 25 sit-ups and 25 push-ups.

By now you may be a little sore and your natural instincts will tell you to let up. But getting in condition means working through soreness, especially in these first few days and weeks.

Monday and Friday are the two most important days of your workout week, because you are either coming off a long weekend or going into a long weekend. What you do on those days will set the tone for what you will accomplish in your upcoming workouts. So if you take it easy because you are a little sore on Friday, Monday it's going to be twice as bad.

A little soreness is natural. It's part of the process of getting in shape. I don't think someone who is getting himself in total condition can do it without some type of muscle discomfort. So don't use soreness as an excuse to slack off. Develop some mental and physical toughness and work through it.

At the same time, let me emphasize that there is a huge difference between natural soreness and an injury. If the pain you are feeling is more than just soreness, or if you have suffered a legitimate injury, don't ignore it. Get it treated. Begin working out again only after a qualified doctor or trainer tells you it is safe to do so.

You may also feel much better than you thought you would at the end of your first week of conditioning: maybe you're not getting winded, your muscles aren't sore, or you feel you should be working harder.

Don't be deluded. You are not yet in condition. Not even close. You haven't been required to push yourself to the maximum, nor should you be at this point.

But consider this week an accomplishment. You are on the right road to getting in condition. You are certainly in better shape than you were before you started. But you have a long way to go before you reach your peak.

Every year, when I complete the first week of the program, I immediately begin to look forward to the second week. I am excited, because I know I've taken the first few steps toward getting in condition. I start preparing for the next step, because I know I'll ask more of myself and expect more from myself.

THE WEEKEND

We're not going to give you specific menus for the weekend. You may not want to adhere to your workout diet on the weekend, and that's okay. But use common sense and don't ruin in two days what you've accomplished in the previous five. Don't load up on fast foods or foods and drinks with a high fat content. Eat sensibly through the weekend. Remember, you are in training. An occasional hamburger or sundae isn't going to hurt you. In fact, that's how I like to reward myself. But if you indulge to excess over the weekend, you are going to pay for it on Monday.

Drink plenty of fluids over the weekend. Fluid replacement doesn't stop because it's Saturday.

Make sure you warm up and stretch each day over the weekend. If you don't, Monday is going to be a nightmare. If you have access to a whirlpool or a Jacuzzi, use it. An alternative is to take a hot bath. If you think you have strained a muscle, get medical attention. If none is immediately available, put ice on the sore area.

Normally this period of transition or easing into condition would not be acceptable to some coaches. But because you haven't done anything for a while and you have a while to go, I think it's wise to get into condition slowly and build gradually.

As the weeks go on, you will see that your training will become more intense. If you've done a good job stretching, your transition will be a smooth one.

W E E K

The emphasis last week was on stretching and flexibility. Though your running was important, its primary purpose was to prepare your muscles for the work you'll be doing beginning this week.

It is important that you continue to maintain your stretching and flexibility exercises in order to advance in the program and reap the benefits from it.

You should continue to concentrate on stretching while we begin to add new phases to the program. This week you will start to build up your stamina by intensifying your running exercises. You will again time yourself and the times you record will become more important because they will serve as a barometer that you can use to measure your progress throughout the program. As the weeks pass, your body will become conditioned to sustained a greater pace and your times should improve.

Later in the program, when you will be in much better shape, your times should not be anywhere near what they are this week. By Week 7, you probably won't even need to time yourself. You'll know whether you're running at a good pace or if you're sloughing off. In the later weeks of the program, I seldom take a clock when I go to the track. I know what I want to accomplish. I know if I'm running hard and putting out my best effort. If I'm not, I don't need a clock to tell me.

After a few weeks, you'll know yourself a lot better. You will know if you're running at a good clip or not. You will know that you're not getting the most out of yourself. That applies even to simple exercises, such as striding a half-mile. The pace you stride a half-mile this week should be slower than the pace you will stride a half-mile five weeks from now.

By the seventh or eighth week of the program, you will probably think that the pace you were running at this week was a leisurely jog.

We are continuing to lay a foundation this week, but at the same time, we are being productive. We cannot have Week 7 without Week 2.

A word of caution: You are not yet close to being in top condition. Don't try to overextend yourself. This program is designed for gradual improvement. You can set yourself back by trying to do too much too soon. Don't cheat yourself on the stretches.

MONDAY

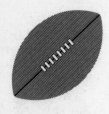

BREAKFAST: You have to start the week with a good breakfast, particularly if you have deviated from your meal plan over the weekend. Start with some orange, apple, or grapefruit juice. Eat some fruit, either half a grapefruit, melon, pineapple, or for variety, cherries. Have a healthful bowl of cold cereal, staying away from those with a high sugar content. Finish with waffles and syrup or honey.

LUNCH: A hot turkey sandwich with whole wheat bread, gravy, and whipped potatoes. Remember to avoid butter. Include a mixed green salad. Drink water or juice with your meal. If you feel like dessert, try some sherbet.

DINNER: Baked chicken with lima beans and/or peas and rice or a baked potato. Don't drink soda with your meal. For dessert, eat a banana or two.

Weigh yourself before going to your workout.
Warm up.

Stretch for 30 to 40 minutes. Try to do the stretches in the same order as you did them last week. You will find that stretching will be easier to complete if you do it in a regular routine, because you won't be spending time wondering what you didn't do.

Pay particular attention to your stretching today, because it is the first day of the workout week and you are in greater danger of pulling a muscle.

When you have completed your stretching, run 2 miles at a faster pace than you ran last week. This sets the tone for the rest of the workout week. You're starting off this week by asking more of yourself than you did last week. It's important to get off to a good start. You don't have to run it at a breakneck pace, but you want to keep track of how fast you run. There's no need to go all out. This isn't a track meet, but you do want to measure your progress.

When you are finished, record your time. Then walk a lap to warm down.

Drink a fluid-replacement beverage every 15 minutes.

Stretch for 30 to 40 minutes.

Finish the day with 25 sit-ups and 25 push-ups.

TUESDAY

BREAKFAST: Begin your day with a glass of juice. If you are growing tired of orange, grapefruit, and apple juice, pineapple, grape, and cranberry juices are tasty and healthful alternatives. Today, have half a cantaloupe. Follow that with pancakes, either plain or blueberry, and syrup. Finish with a sweet roll.

▼

LUNCH: Chicken and rice soup with crackers. Then have a healthy portion of baked sole, with a mixed green salad as a side dish. If you don't feel like eating sole at lunch, substitute a tuna fish sandwich on whole wheat bread. Drink water, juice, or low-fat milk with your lunch. Cherry Jell-O is a good dessert, with or without fruit.

▼

DINNER: Roast turkey with herbed rice, leaf spinach, and/or squash. If neither of those vegetables is to your liking, try broccoli or green beans. Include dinner rolls with your meals and a salad if you wish. Stay away from soda. For dessert, let's stick with the tried-and-true banana.

I realize that at this point in the program our exercises are not very exciting. It's a bit like the first few days of training camp, when the emphasis is on conditioning and some coaches keep the footballs locked in the closet. At times like this, the football season can seem very far away.

But it really isn't. And the way I like to sharpen my concentration during these early weeks of the program is to think back to seasons past and the campaign that lies ahead. I consider the accomplishments I've had and emphasize to myself that I wouldn't have been nearly as successful if not for the hard work I put in during the off-season.

I also think about some of my opponents, who I know are working just as hard as I am. If I slack off now, and I face them later on in the season, they are going to have an edge on me.

One guy I think about in particular is Roger Craig, a three-time Pro Bowl running back with the San Francisco 49ers. I think Roger is a tremendous athlete who is always in top condition. He's a very strong running back you have to contend with from the opening play until the final gun. Roger is the kind of guy who will beat you physically as well as mentally. He's in there every play, always giving 100 percent. He never looks like he's slowing down. I have never seen Roger raise his hand for the coach to take him out of the game.

Playing a guy like Roger Craig should be an inspiration to any defender to be in the best shape he can be, so that he won't be defeated mentally when the game is on the line. It's a big motivation for me. If you need to make a play when Roger is carrying the ball, you don't want to be at a disadvantage. You want to have just as good a chance to make the play as he does for his team.

When Roger is out on the field, you can tell what great shape he's in. He's a horse or a machine that simply will not stop running. Roger is very powerful, with extremely strong legs. And he knows how to use his skills to the maximum. He's not the shiftiest runner, but he has an effective combination of power and elusiveness. He's not the fastest guy in the league either, but you don't need to be when you're the type of runner he is.

Roger is a good open field runner, though he doesn't have the speed of someone like Herschel Walker. At the same time, Walker doesn't have the moves of a Roger Craig. Everyone knows how great Herschel Walker is. But in discussions of contemporary running backs, Roger is often overlooked. I think that he is one of the great running backs to play during my time in the NFL.

He's a very hard guy to tackle, because he is so strong and because he brings his knees up very high when he runs. And he is in such good condition, he never seems to get tired out there.

I have had success in bringing Roger down when I've been able to get to him before he had a full head of steam going. That means getting to him before he gets to the line of scrimmage, and before he picks his hole. Because once he does that, he moves into second gear and it's hard for one man to get him down.

Roger is also tough, because he doesn't give you very good angles from which to tackle him. If he's going through the line of scrimmage, you've got to be right in front of him; he's hard to bring down from the side, because his body movement is so good.

I still have vivid memories of one otherwise unspectacular play from our play-off game against the 49ers following the 1986 season, when we were on our way to the Super Bowl. Roger came through the line of scrimmage and I dove in an attempt to tackle him. But he had those strong legs moving and I just slid off him. I ended up grabbing a leg and waiting for help to arrive.

It is plays like that, and players like Roger Craig, that I think about constantly during these early weeks of my off-season workout program. It makes the start of the season seem a lot closer and it keeps me focused during these strenuous workouts.

You should think about the Roger Craigs in your league and how much speed, strength, and stamina you're going to need to confront them during the season. That will provide you with a lot of extra motivation as you work your way through this program.

Now, let's get on with today's work:

Warm up,
Stretch for 30 to 40 minutes.
Jump rope for at least 30 minutes. If you don't have a jump rope, do some other type of aerobic exercise. But I recommend jumping rope, because it gives you faster, quicker feet. It's an excellent foot-coordination drill. You can use a regular jump, then go side-to-side and up-and-down and you will develop the kind of foot coordination you need in a fast-paced game like football.

WEDNESDAY

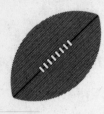

BREAKFAST: Begin your day with a glass of juice. Today we'll have a fruit cocktail, an English muffin with honey, and French toast with syrup.

▼

LUNCH: We'll continue to eat a lot of soup, because it's good energy food. Today, have a bowl of pea soup with crackers. When you've finished that, eat chicken, either baked or chicken à la king, with broccoli. Don't forget your green salad. Drink fluid-replacement beverages.

▼

DINNER: Tonight we'll enjoy baked cod. If you want to add flavoring, use lemon instead of tartar sauce. Eat some peas and cauliflower with that, and be sure to eat your dinner rolls. For dessert, you can stay with a banana or try an orange or pear.

Don't forget to weigh yourself before working out.
Warm up.
Stretch for 30 to 40 minutes.
Run three half-miles, just as you did last week. That means walking a lap between the half-miles. Run a little faster than a jog, time yourself, and record your time. When you are finished, walk a lap to warm down.
Drink a fluid-replacement beverage at regular intervals.
Stretch 30 to 40 minutes.
Finish with 25 sit-ups and 25 push-ups.
Weigh yourself when you get home and drink the proper amount of water-replacement fluids to maintain your weight. You should be weighing yourself before and after every workout.
If you feel muscle tightness or soreness in your legs, do some light stretching during the evening.

THURSDAY

BREAKFAST: Begin the day with a glass of juice. If you're still searching for variety, drink tomato or V-8 juice. Have some honeydew melon or pear halves. Then eat a scrambled egg or two, grits or potatoes, and toast with honey.

▼

LUNCH: Let's begin with chicken soup with noodles or rice. Move on to lasagna with a side dish of green beans. Include a mixed green salad. A reminder: Stay away from fatty, heavy dressings like blue cheese or Thousand Island. Stick to low-fat dressings. Drink the healthful beverages we noted earlier.

▼

DINNER: Tonight we'll have roast pork loin with applesauce. Enjoy some corn on the cob, if it's available. If not, eat mixed vegetables. Complete the main course with a baked potato and dinner rolls. Remember, use little or no butter on either. Add a salad if you like and drink fluid-replacement beverages. Finish your meal with red or green grapes.

Warm up.
Stretch for 45 minutes.
Jump rope for 15 minutes. If you feel like you can do more, jog a half-mile.
Finish your workout day with 25 push-ups and 25 sit-ups.

FRIDAY

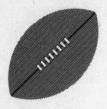

BREAKFAST: Kick off the morning with juice. By now, you should have a pretty good selection to choose from. Then have half a cantaloupe. If they're available, eat strawberries as your fruit of the day. Then eat a bowl of hot cereal and finish the meal with pancakes and syrup.

▼

LUNCH: We want to make sure you have enough carbohydrates, so we'll stick with a pasta lunch. Yesterday, you had spaghetti or fettucine. Today, pick your favorite pasta and enjoy it with tomato or red clam sauce. Include a side dish of cauliflower, as well as a mixed green salad. Drink water, juice, or low-fat milk with your lunch.

▼

DINNER: Baked salmon with lemon wedges. As a side dish, have a sizable portion of Brussels sprouts and wax beans. Include a potato or rice and dinner rolls. Add a salad if you wish and choose from the same drinks you had at lunch. Have a banana or two for dessert.

The program becomes much more strenuous next week, so if you are cheating yourself now at mealtime, you may be playing catch-up a few days from now. Drink plenty of fluid-replacement beverages.

Weigh yourself before working out.
Warm up.
Stretch 30 to 40 minutes.
Run a mile and a half. You should do this at three-quarters of your maximum running speed and maintain a good, steady pace. A mile and a half is not a sprint, but this should be at three-quarters of the speed you would do if you were running a hard mile and a half. I call this striding—you're not jogging and you're not sprinting. Keep a good, constant stride going. Time yourself.
Walk a lap to warm down.
Stretch for 30 to 40 minutes.
Jump rope for 15 minutes.
Finish with 25 sit-ups and 25 push-ups.

Weigh yourself after the workout and replace fluids as needed.

If you are unaccustomed to exercise, you may experience muscle cramps. I have had a problem with cramping and I exercise all the time. They can be caused by a lot of things, one of the most common being dehydration. That's an important reason not to cut back on your fluid intake. Muscle cramps can also be caused by a lack of sodium in the body, particularly in hot weather.

THE WEEKEND

Stretch, preferably an hour each day. Soak in a whirlpool or hot tub.

We have now completed two weeks and, though it is still early, you should be feeling some difference in your physical condition. You should notice improved muscle tone as well as some muscle tightness. There should not be a great deal of discomfort. You will probably have a little soreness.

You should be looking forward to resuming your workouts on Monday.

WEEK 3

This week we are introducing a new phase of our workout program: weight lifting.

Please note: No matter what level you are on, weight training should be closely supervised when you are starting out. You have to have some guidance and guidelines when you are lifting weights, especially when you are younger. Make sure you lift at a facility where you can use the services of an experienced weight coach. Don't try to lift at home without supervision, or any other time you are alone.

Because strength is such an important attribute to have in football, you may wonder why we've waited this long to start lifting weights. The reason is that we didn't want to put much demand on your muscles at one time. If you are not used to heavy exercise, it is important to start slowly and build up gradually. That way you can build up strength and stamina without taxing your body to a great degree. Your body is less likely to break down with a muscle tear or pull or a sore tendon if you proceed carefully.

During the first two weeks, we got your muscles and the rest of your body acclimated to exercise. We didn't want to demand too much of your muscles, because we wanted to get them used to doing some running exercises. And although you don't use the muscles in the upper body in the same manner as you will when you lift weights, they are still being exercised when you run.

We deliberately didn't put too much strain on you, because we

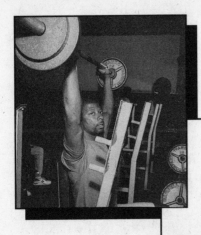

Your weight training should be closely supervised.

wanted you to get accustomed to the routine, as well as an idea of what is going to be expected of you. Unless you are woefully out of shape to begin with, I expect that you got through the first two weeks without much trouble.

If you were almost completely out of shape, then last week's running probably drained you. But you needed to do it to build up stamina so that you can take on another phase of your total body conditioning this week.

It is now time to kick your conditioning program into second gear. This is what I do every off-season. I proceed through the first two weeks exactly as you did, giving my body a chance once again to become comfortable with daily exercise. But in the third week, I start working harder. I begin lifting weights and demanding more of myself. I expect you to do the same.

Lifting weights is just as important as running in preparing for a football season. You can't really maximize your performance without one or the other. You need both. You can be a very fast linebacker, but you'll be at a distinct disadvantage if you're not strong at the point of attack. The strength you acquire in the weight room will come in very handy when you are up against an opponent who is 15 or 20 pounds heavier than you. But if you don't have the endurance to go with the strength, you will run out of gas by halftime.

It takes both strength and stamina to succeed in football. This week, we will work on both.

Weight lifting is not as important in grade school as it is in high school, college, and the pros. But you have to pay very, very close attention to the guidelines set for you.

What will weight training do for you? First, it will help prevent injuries. It gives you the strength to take the pounding that football inflicts on the body.

In addition, it helps you to reach your optimum level of performance and enables you to perform your duties on the field by giving you the strength that running doesn't. To *be* in shape but not *have* any strength is not being in condition to play football. You need your strength on every play, so your weight training should be taken as seriously as your running. You must bring the same discipline and work ethic into the weight room that you bring to the track.

Weight training, when done properly, helps any young person develop physically and gives football players the strength needed to compete in a demanding game. I could not succeed for even the first half of a game against a tight end like New Orleans' John Tice, who is 6 feet 5 inches, 250 pounds, without weight training.

Tice is a very strong and physical opponent. He's the type of guy you have to battle for 60 minutes every time you play him. Tice is a relentless blocker. He's not the kind of player who is going to wear down first, so when I play him, I know I have to be in top condition. If I haven't done my work in the weight room, it's going to hurt me most against a player like Tice.

My college and professional weight programs were different. We do more exercises here in the pros than I did in college. With some players, the opposite is true. Our weight coach on the Giants, Johnny Parker, concentrates on total fitness, total muscle work.

Your coach or instructor will have a prescribed program for you. Different exercises help you do different things on the field. Not all positions on a team do the same type of weight-lifting exercises. Offensive and defensive linemen and tight ends will do more heavy lifting than a running back or defensive back will. A quarterback's program is unlike that of a linebacker.

So please follow your weight instructor's advice. And never lift alone. You always need someone there to spot you. A spotter is someone who can watch you very closely while you are lifting. In case there is a repetition that you can't complete, he can grab the weights.

It is important that you realize you are entering a new phase of your program and that you are putting more demands on your body.

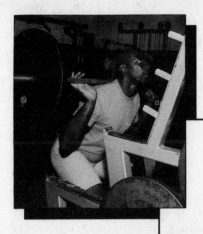

Don't try to lift too much weight.

You will be using a different set of muscles than those you used in the running exercises. You will feel soreness in other parts of your body, so you must consult your weight coach to ensure that you are doing the proper stretches before lifting weights.

No matter what kind of weight program you are following, it should have some type of exercise in which you are using free weights for the upper body and some type of exercise where you are using free weights for the lower body.

Note: If there is no organized weight program that you can get involved in, there are some basic rules you can follow. Don't lift weights that are too light or too heavy for you. It shouldn't be too easy for you to lift the weight, nor should it be too difficult. The weight you choose should be one that allows you to do 4 sets of 10, but it should take some effort. The last three reps of your final set should be a struggle.

If you find after your second set that you are fatigued or arm-weary, lighten up the weight for your last two sets. Do not stop working out. Complete your entire program, even if you have to remove 10 or 15 pounds from what you have been lifting.

A word of advice: Don't exercise by lifting the maximum weight you can handle for any given exercise. If you start out with a very heavy weight, you can cause yourself a lot of pain. You can pull muscles, suffer strains, and throw different parts of your body out of whack; you can also hurt your back. You risk giving yourself a hernia.

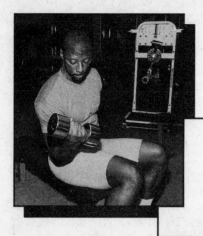

You won't get a good workout if you lift weights that are too light.

Also, starting off with a heavy weight will cause you to tire easily. A good weight is one that allows you to do the suggested number of repetitions. If your program requires you to do six repetitions, a good weight is one in which you can do at least five repetitions. The sixth should require an extra effort, but you shouldn't really have to fight to get the weight up.

You must also lift weights for your lower body, because leg strength helps you stay on your feet when an opponent is trying to knock you down. These exercises can include leg extensions, leg curls, leg press, or squats. I'm a great believer in squats, but I think you should listen to the recommendations of your weight instructor.

Weight lifting is just like running in that you have to warm up first. You should stretch before you do the different weight-lifting exercises. Of particular importance when lifting weights for the upper body are stretches that strengthen the shoulders. And leg stretches are very important before doing lower body lifting.

You should consult with your weight coach to find out what stretches you should do to maximize your performance in the weight room. It is important that your back, shoulders, and hips are loose before you lift weights.

I then start by lifting light weights and I recommend that you do the same. If you are going to bench press, start by lifting 20 percent of the maximum weight you can handle. Once the blood is flowing and your muscles are warm, work your way up to the weight you will use for the majority of this workout. I've used this system with success since the tenth grade. Along the way, I've seen other players suffer serious injuries because they didn't warm up before lifting or they tried to lift weights with an improper technique.

Make sure you don't work with a weight that is too light. If you do, you won't get anything out of the exercise. But you can use a light weight to warm up. That will get the blood flowing in your muscles and prepare you for lifting the heavier weights.

It is also important to remember that muscle is weight. Whenever you gain weight, you have to compensate so that your body can easily carry the additional muscle. If you simply add muscle, but don't run, you're going to be big. But you will be a football failure because you can't move: you have to do the necessary running so you can carry the extra weight. If you feel sluggish running, lose a little weight so you can run more easily.

I will now detail several of my weight-lifting exercises. You may wind up using all of them, some of them, or almost none of them. Your weight-lifting instructor will lay out a program for you and some of these exercises will probably be included. But he knows what your needs and limitations are. Use the following synopsis as a guide, but please follow your instructor's advice.

There's an old saying on our team that you can look like Tarzan and play like Jane. Do the exercises that will help you play better, not the exercises that are going to make you look better.

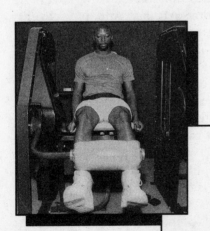

Make sure you get plenty of rest.

MONDAY

BREAKFAST: We're beginning an important week here, so make sure you eat right. Make sure you have a glass of juice, as well as some fruit. Half a grapefruit, melon, or apricots are good. Let's have some hot cereal and French toast with syrup. If you're still looking for extra energy, eat an English muffin with honey.

▼

LUNCH: Ravioli, preferably cheese, with peas as a side dish. If you're still stuffed from breakfast, try a seafood salad sandwich on whole wheat bread. Either way, make sure you have your mixed green salad. Drink water or juice with your meal.

▼

DINNER: We'll stick with Italian food tonight. Make your main course veal parmigiana with a side dish of brown rice. Add some carrots to your meal, plus dinner rolls. Stay away from soda and other sweets. For dessert, try a plum or two.

Warm up.

Stretch for 30 to 40 minutes. If you did not stretch much over the weekend, take extra care when you do so today. And pay careful attention to your upper body stretches today, because you will be using those muscles more now than you did in the first two weeks.

Jump rope for 10 minutes.

Run a mile and a half and time yourself. Try to complete the distance 10 seconds faster than you ran it last Friday.

Walk a lap to warm down, then stretch again.

This would be the time I would do my weight lifting. You may decide to do it earlier in the day, before you run. I will leave that up to you. Your decision will probably depend on the accessibility you have to a track and weight room, your schedule, and your personal preference.

It doesn't matter in what order you do your running and lifting. What is important is that you not cheat yourself in either area.

To compete in the NFL, I have to continually work in the weight room. If I didn't, my upper body and legs would grow weaker, and if I didn't remedy the situation, I'd get pushed around on the field. I guard against that by spending as much time lifting weights as I do running.

Upper Body

My weight exercises are very basic. For the upper body I start with a *bench press*, which utilizes an arm motion used at every position on the football field. You are pushing something away from your body, such as a charging blocker like Luis Sharpe of the Phoenix Cardinals. A bench press builds up the shoulders, arms, and chest. It's almost like an upside-down push-up with weights. You lie on your back and push the weight up, then slowly bring it down. A bench press simulates explosion with the arms and chest. You are pushing the weights as you would push an opponent on the field, with a thrusting motion.

Do 4 sets of 10 at a weight that is comfortable. Take at least two or three minutes between sets, but not more than seven or eight minutes.

The bench press is in the same weight-training family as the military press and the incline press. When doing a bench press you are lying down. In a *military press*, which is very similar to an

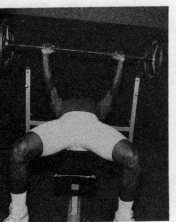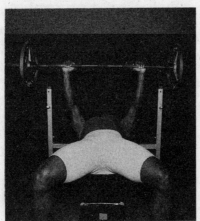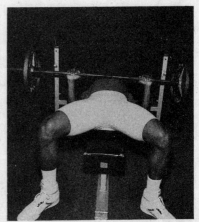

The *bench press* is an excellent weight-lifting exercise because it builds muscle while simulating the arm motions used on the football field.

incline press, you are sitting in an upright position; this further individualizes the muscles. The *incline press* has you sitting at an angle. Each press you do in different positions develops different muscles in the shoulder or chest area. You should do all three or one muscle is going to become weaker than the other muscles. Your shoulders may develop, but at the expense of weak biceps. Sometimes you may not even know the difference, but it is better to be safe than sorry.

The *military press* is like a bench press, except it is done sitting upright. It develops muscles that would be ignored by the bench press.

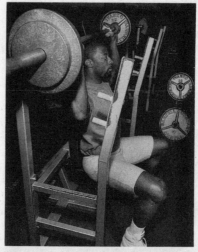
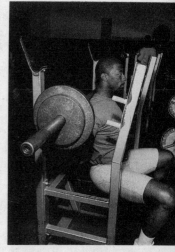
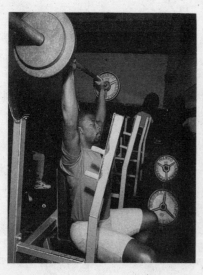
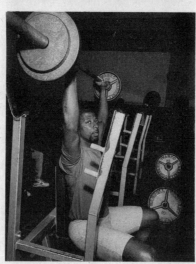
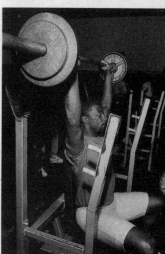

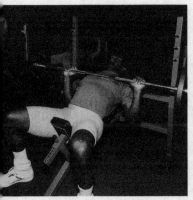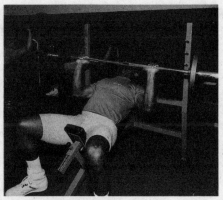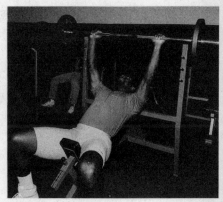

The *incline press* is the cousin to the bench press and the military press. Failure to do all three could result in some underdeveloped shoulder and arm muscles.

Bench pressing is important in any weight workout. I do 6 sets of 8 repetitions apiece. I start at about 135 to 140 pounds and gradually work my way up to 285 to 295. The vast majority of the readers of this book will not work with such heavy weight. And I suggest you limit yourself to 4 sets of 10. But it is crucial that you follow the idea of building up the amount of weight you lift, rather than lifting the heavier weight at the beginning of the workout.

The incline press is similar to the bench press, except that the bench is at a 45-degree angle. It further isolates the muscles you work on, primarily the shoulder and deltoid muscles. The amount of weight I lift is not as great, but I do the same number of sets.

Another weight exercise is the *dumbbell bench press*, in which I have a dumbbell in each hand. I'll start with a warm-up set of 10 reps at 40 pounds. Then I will increase the weight in 10-pound increments until I have 50 pounds in each hand. I also do a *dumbbell military press* and a *dumbbell incline press*.

Power cleans are also part of my regular workout. They simulate the explosion motion from top to bottom. With a power clean, you start with the weight below the knees and bring it all the way up to your chest. I do 4 or 5 sets, with fewer reps. I start at about 135 pounds and have gone as high as 335 pounds.

A lot of weight coaches don't believe in curls, including *dumbbell curls* and *barbell curls*. They're basically body-builder's exercises, but football players can also benefit from them. I do curls to improve the strength of the triceps and biceps muscles in my arms.

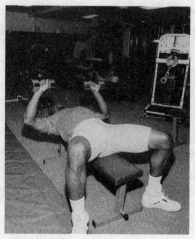 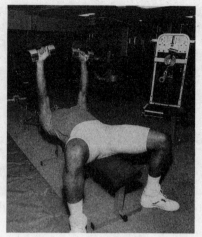 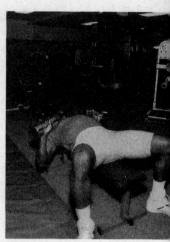

The *dumbbell bench press* allows you to work on each arm separately or both of them at the same time.

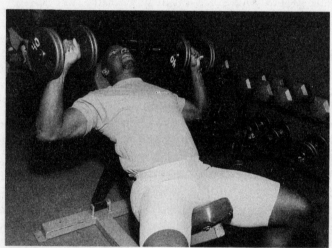

The *dumbbell incline press* is an excellent exercise for building up arm muscles.

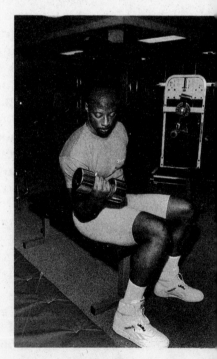

Although curls are used primarily by body-builders, I do them because I believe they benefit football players. This *dumbbell curl* builds up the biceps and triceps.

Curls do not have to be a major part of your program. Much of the reason that athletes like to do them is for looks, because they make the arms bigger. And bigger is sometimes not better. You want real strength, not good looks.

There are also some isometric exercises that I have found to be very important for the neck. This does not include the actual lifting of weights, but pushing against resistance. They are done in three or four basic positions.

While you are lying down on your stomach with your head hanging over the bench, your teammate or lifting partner should lightly place his hands on the back of your head. You should then try to move your head against the pressure he is applying. When you complete that, have him place his hands on the side, front, and then the other side of your head.

These exercises give you a stronger neck, which helps prevent pinched nerves and other neck injuries.

Lower Body

The number one exercise for leg explosion—and it's not one of my favorites, but I have to do it—is a *squat*. They are universally used throughout football. Squats are great for building up your legs, particularly the hamstrings and quadriceps, which help a player run faster and longer. They also build up your butt. A strong rear helps you avoid getting pushed around on a football field, because it gives you tremendous leverage.

I recommend you do *back squats,* in which the weight bar is resting behind your neck on your shoulders. You have to keep your back in an upright position. The best way to do that is to find a spot on the ceiling and focus on it. You then squat down as far as the seat of a chair, or below. Your coach will tell you exactly how far to go. Once you're down, you have to bring the weight back up. When you do, you take the pressure off your back and shoulders and try to use all leg power.

This is a very, very delicate exercise. It must be done properly and it must be done with the correct amount of weight. If it is done incorrectly, it could easily lead to back and knee problems. Using equipment such as knee wraps and a weight belt can help prevent those kinds of injuries.

Some players can't do squats because they have bad backs. The amount of weights used in squats naturally puts pressure on the

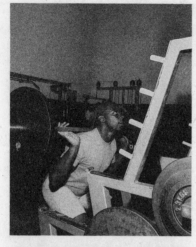
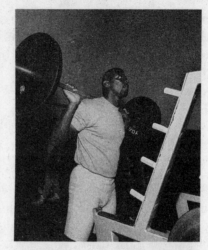

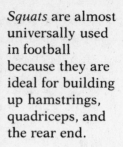
Squats are almost universally used in football because they are ideal for building up hamstrings, quadriceps, and the rear end.

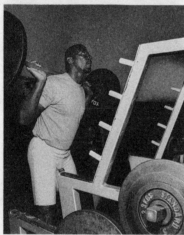
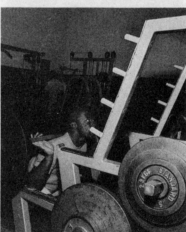

back. If you absolutely can't do squats, there are leg press, leg curl, and leg extension machines that simulate squats without putting the same pressure on the back. The machines can't match the same explosion in your legs that the squats give you. But they will build up the muscles in the hamstrings and quadriceps.

With a *leg press*, you lie on your back and lift the weight. I might begin with six 45-pound Nautilus plates, doing 2 sets of 10. As the weight increases, the reps decrease. If I get it up to 12 plates, I may do 2 sets of 5. When I do *leg extensions*, in which I lift the weight with my legs while I am sitting down, I do 2 sets of 10 reps with 12

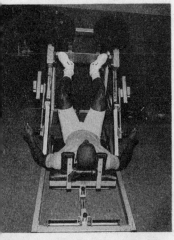
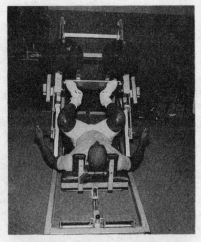
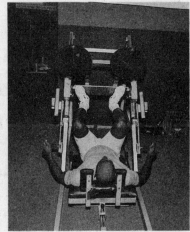
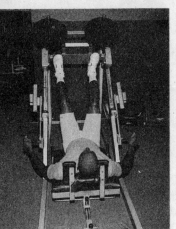
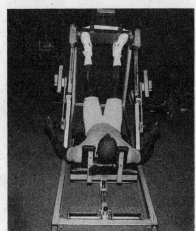

Leg extensions are demanding exercises that help build muscles in both the upper and lower parts of the legs. Be careful that you don't try to push too much weight.

to 15 plates. For *leg curls,* in which I am lying on my stomach, I use 8 to 10 plates.

I also recommend doing *calf raises* which help strengthen the muscles in the lower part of the leg. Stand straight with your hands on your hips. Push up on your toes and hold for a count of 3. Repeat 10 to 15 times. It is important that you work on building up all the muscles in your legs during the course of a workout.

On the Giants, we have an exercise we call *good morning.* I sit on the very edge of the bench, with my legs straight and fully extended, and rest a bar with very light weight on my shoulders. You may

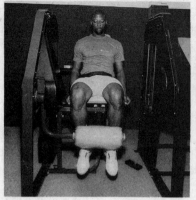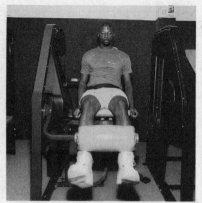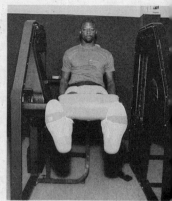

Just as a military press exercises different muscles than the bench press, *leg extensions* enable you to build up different muscles than the leg press.

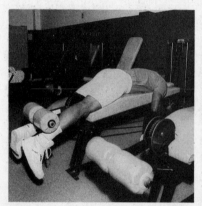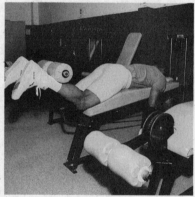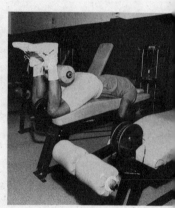

Leg curls will probably be your most challenging lower body weight exercise. Start with weights that allow you to move your legs freely and build up gradually.

need no more than a broomstick. I then bend down and come back up very slowly. The good mornings both stretch and strengthen the hamstrings. Once you have been doing this for a while, you will have to increase the weight, but it will never be anything too heavy.

We have just covered the basic exercises for football, using both free weights and machines. Your instructor may have several more he wants you to work on. You will probably need some of the individual exercises, such as a dumbbell incline using alternating arms. That exercise singles out the muscles and helps each shoulder individually. It is often better than using a full-length bar, because by alternating arms you can't compensate when one shoulder is weaker than another. They both have to do the work.

I also use what I call *natural weight training*. This includes push-ups, pull-ups, and sit-ups. You have already done some push-ups and sit-ups, probably just the way you learned to do them from your dad or your phys. ed. teacher at school. In a moment, I will discuss the different kinds of push-ups and sit-ups I want you to start doing.

For younger players, who may not be ready to use weights or have access to a weight room, the natural weight training can serve as an excellent alternative. They can also be additional assets that you get in the weight room. But they are so beneficial I make sure to do them almost every time I work out.

By pushing natural weight, you are further strengthening muscles that the weights helped you develop. They are like isometric exercises, because you are pushing against your own resistance.

Any weight coach will tell you that a push-up cannot simulate a bench press. But I look at that in reverse. A bench press can't simulate a push-up, which works on muscles a bench press may not completely challenge.

I use different types of push-ups. The most basic is the *military push-up*. The hands are flat on the ground about shoulder width

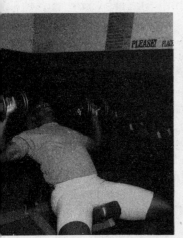
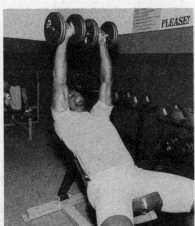
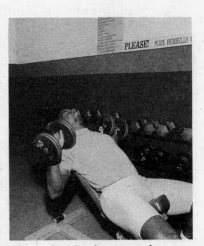

By using the *dumbbell incline*, you will be able to work on individual arm and shoulder muscles more easily than with the presses. Work on your arms individually and together.

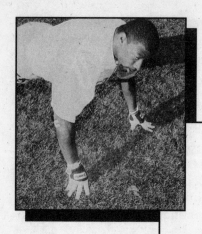

Fingertip push-ups are the hardest to do, but they are the most beneficial.

apart. Keep your back straight and parallel to the ground. If you hunch your back so you don't have to go down as far, then you are cheating. You should go down and come up slowly. To qualify as a complete push-up, you should touch your chin to the ground. These push-ups develop the hands, wrists, and upper body.

The type of push-up that may be the hardest, but most beneficial, is the *fingertip push-up*. They are done just like the military push-ups, except that you should be on your fingertips instead of the palms of your hands. These are very good for football players to do, because they strengthen the fingers, hands, and wrists.

With both of those kinds of push-ups, you should vary your hand position. Do a set of 15 with your hands about shoulder width apart, then keep moving them in until they are almost touching each other.

Sit-ups are good for strengthening the abdominal muscles as well as the back. Those are critical areas of the body, because they connect the upper body and the lower body. If they are weak, there will be a chance for the muscles in the other parts of the body to become weak also. If you pull abdominal or back muscles, you will quickly find that there is not a lot you can do, except wait for them to heal. If your stomach or back is hurting, you will be very limited.

The other natural weight exercises are the *pull-ups* or *chin-ups*, which are really the same thing. You will need a bar that hangs a little higher than the top of your head. Grab it with both hands. You then have to pull your own weight up against gravity, and lift

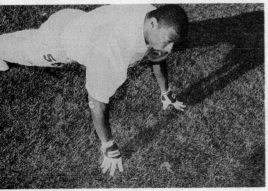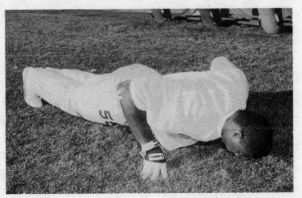

Fingertip push-ups are challenging but beneficial because they help strengthen your hands, wrists, and fingers.

yourself until your chin is above the bar. If you can do this 10 times, you are doing very well. These are basic arm and shoulder exercises. They are also excellent exercises for strengthening your hands and grip, because you have to hang on and pull your body up.

I don't like to do pull-ups, but I know they are very helpful. The main reason I don't like doing them is that I weigh more than 200 pounds. But by pulling my own weight, I have really built up my arm strength.

Just as you do with push-ups, you should vary the width of your hand position on the bar. Start with a wide grip and gradually move it in.

It is important that weight lifting stay a part of your training ritual at least three times a week. Anything less and your strength may slip, which will surely carry over to your performance on the field. You will be getting the running you need during football practice. If you're not satisfied, you can always do more. But you have to maintain your strength or you will be dragging at the end of the season.

Think of it as maintenance work. You won't be lifting as hard as you did during this program, but you will be lifting to maintain your strength over the course of the season. You do that to protect yourself against injury and maintain your level of play. If you get weaker, your performance starts to slack off.

On the Giants, we work out in the weight room two days a week during the season. That doesn't include the very light workout we have at the beginning of the week, right after a game. The early-week lifting session is done primarily to work out muscle soreness that we naturally feel after a game.

You will also feel sore after a game. But if you keep up with your weight lifting, you will get rid of it a lot faster.

No matter what position you play, you are going to need both running and weight training. Each weight program is tailored for a specific position. But my running program is useful to everyone.

Another important point to remember is that, like running, don't try to accomplish everything in the weight room in one day. Just as we didn't start out with 100-yard sprints, don't move into your weight work full blast. You have time to reach your strength goals, just as you have time in the other phases of this program. Follow your weight instructor's advice, because he has a good idea of what your specific needs and limitations are.

Don't forget to stretch before and after lifting weights. It is just as important as the stretching you do before and after you run.

Another important point to remember is that you must replace your fluids. Between exercises, be sure to drink a fluid-replacement beverage. After eating, try to wait two hours before beginning your workout. That will give the food sufficient time to digest.

TUESDAY

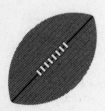

BREAKFAST: Start with a glass of juice and some fruit. Still searching for variety? Try blueberries. They're delicious. Then we'll have two or three scrambled eggs with potatoes or grits, and toast, muffin, or a bagel.

▼

LUNCH: Treat yourself today with something we all like: pizza. Choose any topping you want, including sausage, pepperoni, mushrooms, or whatever else you like on your pizza. Don't forget a green salad and fluid-replacement beverages.

▼

DINNER: With a big day coming up tomorrow, we'll turn to another old favorite, spaghetti and meat balls. Include some hot mixed vegetables as a side dish, as well as dinner rolls. For dessert, let's eat some green grapes or a peach.

Warm up. Don't start taking this for granted just because you've been working out for more than two weeks. Everything in my program has a purpose. It's important to get off to a good start every day. Warm up until you break a sweat.

Stretch for 30 to 40 minutes. Do something that gets you moving, whether it's a half-mile jog or jumping rope for 15 minutes. You don't have to push yourself; you're just doing something to get your muscles working, break and sweat, and work some soreness out of your body. Don't overextend yourself by trying to do too much. Stick to the program.

You will probably experience a little more muscle soreness because you used different muscles while weight lifting yesterday. Use a whirlpool if possible to work out some of that soreness. If you don't have access to a whirlpool, soak in a hot bath.

While you're soaking, think of what you want to accomplish during the football season. Imagine the great things you want to do. Try to picture what certain opponents may try to do when they face you.

That's how I spend a lot of my time in the off-season. I think about some of the players I know I will be up against. And since this is the week we start weight lifting, some of the stronger blockers—including the ones that like to hold—that I will be up against. As you might suspect, a lot of holding goes on at the line of scrimmage during a pro football game.

The best blockers are not the best holders. Some of the better blockers are good holders, but I think the guys that just come out and hold have no confidence in their blocking abilities. One of the tricks a good blocker and holder uses is grabbing a defensive player, getting him close to his body, and then trying to move him. It's a ploy the officials often have trouble spotting.

I don't enjoy going up against a player who only wants to hold me, instead of trying to block me. One of them is Damone Johnson, the tight end for the Los Angeles Rams. He weighs 250 pounds and all he wants to do is hold. We've played the Rams several times and

Johnson never tried to move me off the ball. He just held me and whichever way I wanted to go, he'd let me go. He'd just keep holding and pushing, trying to get me away from the play.

It can be an effective block, but it's sometimes very risky, because the officials can penalize you.

You can combat moves like that with strength and fast hands. That's where all of your weight room work comes in. You have to get your hands on the inside of his. You extend your arms so he won't have the outside of your shoulder pads to grab.

It takes strength to do that and to beat a persistent holder. You gain that strength in the weight room.

WEDNESDAY

BREAKFAST: Kick off with a glass of your favorite juice. Let's mix up the fruit today and have a fruit cocktail. Then we'll eat pancakes, either plain or blueberry. If you'd like, you can also have a bagel, muffin, or toast.

LUNCH: Baked scrod with green beans. I enjoy this meal, but I know it may not appeal to many of you. If not, try a tuna fish sandwich on whole wheat bread. Eat a mixed green salad and if that doesn't fill you up, eat a bowl of tomato soup. Drink water or juice. Top off your lunch with a bowl of Jell-O, with or without fruit.

DINNER: I've got another treat for you. For our main course tonight, we'll enjoy prime ribs of beef. Make sure it is lean. Cut away all the excess fat. With that, have some stir-fry vegetables. Fry them in olive oil and don't put butter on them. You should also eat a baked potato or oven-browned potatoes. Don't forget the dinner rolls and fluid-replacement drinks. For dessert, eat a red or green apple.

Weigh yourself before working out. Remember to drink fluids throughout your workout.

Stretch for 30 to 40 minutes. Jog a lap around the track. Stretch again for 5 minutes.

Run three separate half-miles for time. Walk a lap in between the running. Your goal should be to improve your time by 10 seconds over the best you achieved in Week 2. Record your time.

Warm down, then stretch for 30 minutes. Finish with 25 sit-ups and 25 push-ups. Make sure you take the time to warm down after every session.

Lift weights. I will continue to list lifting weights at the end of a workout day. As I've said previously, you can lift before you run. You should gauge which is better for you according to your time frame, daily schedule, and access to a weight room or track. If you don't have a lot of time in the afternoon, I would suggest lifting weights first and then running.

You should not lift weights immediately after you run, or, if you do them in the reverse order, do not head to the track as soon as you leave the weight room. Take at least 30 to 40 minutes to allow your body to recuperate. During that recuperation period, you can stretch and drink fluid-replacement beverages.

THURSDAY

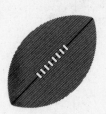

BREAKFAST: Start off with a glass of juice and a grapefruit half. Then have a bowl or two of healthful cold cereal, making sure to avoid those with added sugar. Complement that with an English muffin and honey.

LUNCH: Have a bowl of vegetable soup or clam chowder with crackers. Then eat a turkey club on whole wheat bread with a side dish of potato salad. Of course, we will also have green salad and healthy beverages.

DINNER: Tonight we'll eat baked flounder with rice and mixed vegetables. Remember to drink water or juice with your meal. For dessert, eat a pear, peach, or banana.

Warm up.
Stretch for 30 minutes.
Jump rope for 15 minutes.
Do 25 sit-ups and 25 push-ups.

Now that you are fully into the program, including weight lifting, you may want to supplement your diet with vitamins, protein supplements, mineral supplements, amino acids, or something else you believe will help you get bigger, stronger, and faster in a hurry. You might be especially tempted to try them if you are trying to put on weight for the football season.

I don't think you should, especially at a young age. Ronnie Barnes believes strongly that eating well-balanced meals that increase your calorie intake is the only proper way to increase your weight and prepare your body for the physical challenges it faces in a program like this.

The best way to get all the vitamins, minerals, carbohydrates, and proteins is with a balanced diet. If you eat smart, you should not need to supplement between or after meals.

FRIDAY

BREAKFAST: Begin your final big day this week with a glass of juice and a fruit cocktail. Follow that with waffles and honey. Have a sweet roll or English muffin if you feel you need more.

LUNCH: We'll introduce a new dish today by starting with a bowl of cream of celery soup. We need some carbohydrates to get us through the weekend, so we'll eat a plate of stuffed pasta shells and a mixed green salad. Drink water or juice and complete your lunch with Jell-O, if you wish.

DINNER: Tonight we'll have chicken parmigiana with fresh carrots and mashed potatoes. Add a salad if you like and don't forget the dinner rolls.

Drink water or juice. You can deviate from the norm at dessert time. Have a bowl of ice milk and strawberries. Ice milk is better than ice cream because it is less fattening. If you prefer, eat a bunch of red grapes.

Weigh yourself before working out.

Warm up.

Stretch for 30 to 40 minutes.

Run a mile and a half and try to better Monday's time by 5 seconds. This will give you an indication whether you have improved both your stamina and your endurance, which these longer running exercises are designed to do. Record your time.

Drink fluid-replacement beverages at regular intervals.

Walk a lap. Then stride a half-mile.

Warm down and stretch.

Do your weight work.

Do 25 sit-ups and 25 push-ups.

THE WEEKEND

Warm up, stretch, and soak. Take extra care with muscles that may be sore because of this week's new work. Maintain your good dietary habits.

I don't think you should overextend yourself at this point. We still have a long way to go. But if you want to do more over the weekend than warm up and stretch, jog a mile or a mile and a half. Do some sit-ups and push-ups. But don't get yourself too tired, because you want to be ready to go on Monday.

WEEK 4

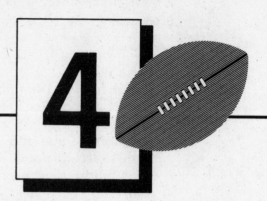

You should be seeing some pretty obvious signs of improvement by now as we approach the halfway point of the program. Unless you haven't been following instructions, your condition should be almost 50 percent better than when you started three weeks ago. It's time to start demanding more of your body. And after what you've asked it to do the last three weeks, your body should respond in a positive manner.

This week, we're going to start emphasizing quality more than quantity. In order to get better time, we are going to use some shorter exercises and cut down on the number of repetitions we ask you to do. Now is the time to demand more of yourself, to build self-esteem regarding your physical condition.

Getting in shape can be very demoralizing. You often have nothing to feel good about, because your body hurts so badly. You might not be seeing results as quickly as you would like. Some evenings, you may feel miserable. I do, too. It's all part of reaching your ultimate goal. When you are hurting or struggling, you have to think about how much better you will feel later on in the program.

It may seem relative, but it is better to feel awful in the first two weeks of the program than in the last two weeks, when it really counts. It takes time to get in shape. If you put in only a lazy effort in Weeks 1 through 8 and you think you're going to accomplish everything you want in the final two weeks, you are going to be in

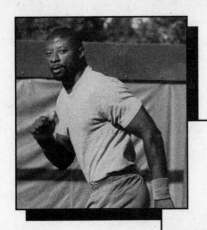

If you take shortcuts now, you won't be in shape to play the game.

for an unpleasant surprise: you will find yourself pulling muscles and straining muscles. You are only getting yourself up to do half a job if you prepare with half an effort. On the football field, doing half a job will result in you getting hurt. If you're lucky, it will net you a seat on the bench. It will never enable you to reach your goals.

If you take shortcuts now, you won't be able to make demands on your body when you need it to respond at the critical juncture of a game. You may get the response you're looking for in the first three quarters. But by the end of the game, when you need it most, you won't have it, because you didn't pay the price before the season. The laziness you bring to your workout today could easily translate into a failed effort on the football field during the season. I would almost guarantee it.

With that in mind, we turn up our efforts a notch this week. We are beginning to narrow our scope and our focus. You should realize by now that there's a lot of potential that we are capable of bringing out of ourselves. And now is the time to start doing it.

It's pretty difficult early in the program to demand certain things of yourself or to set specific goals, when you're feeling miserable and trying to get into shape. But by being in shape, you can set your goals on the things you want to accomplish in the game of football. That's the way I feel about tackling this program every year.

The first couple of weeks, I'm trying to get in shape. By Week 4, I'm starting to feel good about myself. My body is starting to look and feel like a real football player's body. I increasingly think about game situations and what I want to accomplish in football. I want to be able to do certain things and my body is telling me that I can't. So I keep working.

I expect you to do the same.

MONDAY

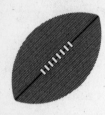

BREAKFAST: We'll begin the week with a glass of juice and a cantaloupe or honeydew melon half. Then have a bowl or two of hot cereal, along with an English muffin and honey. Finish off the meal with a fruit Danish.

LUNCH: Start off with a bowl of navy bean soup with crackers. Then eat a turkey or seafood salad sandwich on the bread of your choice, as well as a green salad. Drink water or juice with your meal and have a small portion of sherbet if you desire.

DINNER: Tonight we'll eat a baked half chicken with a baked potato, cranberry sauce, and mixed vegetables. Our dessert tonight will be a banana or two.

Weigh yourself before working out.
Warm up.
Stretch for 30 to 40 minutes.
Jump rope for 10 minutes.
Run three half-miles. Try to improve your time by 5 seconds over the times you had last Wednesday. Walk a lap in between your half-miles. Five seconds is a lot to ask for in just five days when you're running a half-mile. But, as we said, it is time to demand more from your body. It's time to step up our production. Getting in shape is not easy.

Jump rope for 10 more minutes. Don't forget to drink the fluid-replacement beverages.

Warm down and stretch for 30 minutes.

Do your weight work. You may feel tired, but it is important to push yourself. If you get in the habit of giving up now, it will carry over to the football field.

Finish with 25 sit-ups and 25 push-ups.

Drink fluids to replace lost weight.

TUESDAY

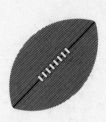

BREAKFAST: We'll begin today with a glass of juice and a grapefruit half. Then we'll have French toast and syrup with grilled ham slices, plus an English muffin or toast with honey.

▼

LUNCH: Chicken soup with rice or noodles, followed by macaroni and cheese, with a side dish of cauliflower or peas, as well as a tossed salad. Drink water, juice, or low-fat milk with your lunch. Complete the meal with a bowl of Jell-O.

▼

DINNER: Our main dish this evening will be fillet of sole, along with rice, zucchini, and rolls or cornbread. Drink healthful beverages, and for dessert, try apples or plums.

Warm up.

Stretch for 45 minutes.

Jump rope for at least 10 minutes in two 5-minute intervals. Rest for 2 minutes in between your jump rope sets.

Jumping rope is an excellent aerobic exercise. It enables you to work up a sweat without the strain of running. It provides a nice change of pace between our heavy workout days. But I don't jump rope just to fill time on my lighter workout days. I think jumping

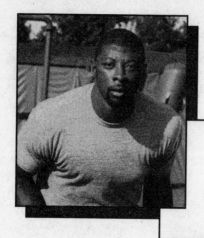

Jumping rope is an excellent way to develop quick feet.

rope is essential for many football players, because it helps you develop quick feet.

Running backs, defensive backs, linebackers, wide receivers, offensive linemen . . . players at just about every position need foot quickness to excel.

I jump rope regularly to improve quickness of foot and foot coordination. The faster you can jump rope, the faster your feet will become. Jumping rope is an exercise used by the vast majority of professional boxers, because of the improvement it makes in their footwork. It can do the same thing for you.

Finish with 25 sit-ups and 25 push-ups.

By now, you may be wondering why I put myself through this every year. It's simple. I want to have a long career in the NFL. The only way to do that is by staying healthy. And you don't stay healthy in professional football if you're not in top condition. Of course, beginning in top shape doesn't guarantee you will have a long career. But it definitely increases your chances.

I have a great deal of respect for players that have been around a long time because it's not easy to have a lengthy career in the NFL. Anyone who does it has to be doing something right. If a longtime veteran is still accomplishing great feats, then you have to respect him.

Look at Joe Montana, whom I have faced many times. The 1990 season was his twelfth, but he was still playing with the enthusiasm of a rookie and the poise and grace of the veteran that he is. In a Monday night game against us late in the 1989 season, he completed 27 of 33 passes, including three for touchdowns, and did not have one intercepted. The 49ers beat us that night, 34–24.

Montana is that good after so long because he keeps his body in great condition. I think that's the key for any player who survives in the NFL for a long time. The guys who play the longest certainly have a little luck on their side, but they're taking care of their bodies and they're making their own breaks. They create situations where they can play longer.

That's what I'm trying to do and I hope you learn how to do it on your level of football.

WEDNESDAY

BREAKFAST: Start your workout day with a glass of juice and some fruit cocktail. Then move on to a plate of waffles and syrup, plus toast or an English muffin with honey.

▼

LUNCH: We'll push up one of our dinner favorites and have spaghetti and meat sauce for lunch today. With that we'll have a tossed salad and rolls, as well as a good fluid-replacement drink. If you want dessert, try sherbet or Jello-O.

▼

DINNER: Fish is a very good workout food, so we'll eat some for the second night in a row. Tonight we'll make it swordfish, which is very tasty. Along with that, have some rice or broccoli or zucchini. Remember not to drink soda. For dessert, have a banana or peach.

Weigh yourself before working out.
Warm up.
Stretch for 30 to 40 minutes.

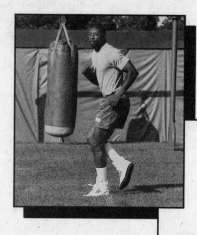

Good footwork is important at every position.

Run a half-mile that is at least as fast as the fastest half-mile you ran on Monday.

Do three 440-yard runs. These should seem a little easier than running a half-mile, because the distance is a little shorter. But you shouldn't be able to breeze through it. At a minimum, you should be able to run a 440 thirty seconds faster than you ran Monday's half-mile. Push yourself. Don't slack off.

The 440s are an indication that we are starting to build up to the sprint work, though I still classify the 440s as endurance work.

Make sure you drink fluids regularly.

Warm down and stretch for 30 minutes.

Do your weight work.

Finish the day with 25 sit-ups and 25 push-ups.

Drink fluids to replace lost weight.

If your muscles are feeling unusually sore after running the 440s, do some light stretching this evening.

THURSDAY

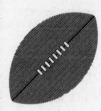

BREAKFAST: Begin with a glass of juice and half a cantaloupe. Then eat a bowl or two of honey-sweetened hot cereal, with toast, a bagel, or an English muffin. Eat extra bread if you're not filled up.

▼

LUNCH: Vegetable soup with crackers, followed by barbecued chicken. Make sure it's barbecued and not fried. Include a mixed green salad and a roll or two with your meal and eat a bowl of cherry Jello-O for dessert. Drink water or fruit juice.

▼

DINNER: Tonight we'll try a new dish, a veal chop. Make sure it is very lean. Have a baked potato with that, as well as cauliflower and green peas. Make sure you also eat rolls or French bread. Drink beverages that are good for you. Our dessert tonight will be grapes or plums.

Warm up.
Stretch for 45 minutes.
Jump rope for at least 10 minutes at 5-minute intervals. Rest for 2 minutes between your jump rope sets.
Do 25 sit-ups and 25 push-ups.
Do some evening stretching if you feel the need. Remember, there is no such thing as too much stretching.

FRIDAY

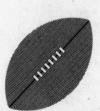

BREAKFAST: Begin the day with a glass of your favorite juice and half a grapefruit. Then have two scrambled eggs with grits or potatoes, plus an English muffin or toast with honey.

▼

LUNCH: We'll eat a bowl of Manhattan clam chowder and crackers, along with a turkey sandwich (two if you desire) on whole wheat bread. Make sure you have a tossed salad and proper fluids. If you'd like dessert, stick with Jell-O or sherbet.

▼

DINNER: Broiled scallops—again, stay away from fried foods—plus green beans, a baked potato, and dinner rolls. Since it's the end of the week, treat yourself to a bowl of ice milk or low-fat frozen yogurt for dessert.

Weigh yourself before working out.
Warm up.
Stretch for 30 to 40 minutes.
Run a mile and a half. Strive to get a good time. Make sure you run at a good pace. This should be your fastest pace to date. Put a little extra effort into achieving that. Record your time.
Do three 440-yard runs. Try to run them at a faster pace than you did on Wednesday.
Warm down and stretch 30 minutes.
Drink fluids regularly.
Do your weight work.
Finish with 30 sit-ups and 30 push-ups.
Drink fluids to replace lost weight.

THE WEEKEND

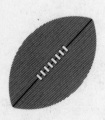

Warm up, stretch, and soak each day. Pay careful attention to your upper body stretches. You have been lifting weights for two weeks now and can probably feel a difference in your strength. In some or most of your exercises, you have probably increased the weight.

But you want to make sure you don't lose flexibility as you add weight. For that reason, make sure you just don't go through the motions when you are doing your upper body stretches. If you don't feel you are loose enough, repeat the sequence. Your extra bulk and strength won't do you much good if you can't use it on the football field. And to be successful there, you have to be flexible.

A player I've gone up against many times who has both strength and flexibility—not to mention quickness and football smarts—is Luis Sharpe, a tackle with the Phoenix Cardinals. Luis is one of the outstanding players on that team. I know, because I come into contact with him a great deal.

He has some characteristics that are common in offensive linemen. Sharpe is 280 pounds, but he has very good feet; they're extremely quick compared to most linemen I have faced in the league. Sharpe is just a great athlete. Even Lawrence Taylor has had trouble with him over the years because Sharpe moves so well.

I think Sharpe is an extremely well rounded offensive tackle. He adjusts well to fakes because his feet and movement allow him to.

In a game we played against the Cardinals in Giants Stadium on September 24, 1989, I tried to beat Sharpe around the corner on an outside speed rush. He made a nice adjustment and I didn't get close to the quarterback. When I got back to the huddle, I said to myself that since he was moving out there that far outside, I could start out in that direction and then spin inside toward the quarterback.

Well, the next chance I got I put my little plan into action. I started rushing up the field on the outside, then spun in toward the middle. Sharpe adjusted perfectly. It was just as though I had never taken him outside in the first place, or that he had read my mind. He was never fooled.

That's very unusual for an offensive lineman. With most of them, if they play you for one move, they are looking for it the rest of the game. If you adjust to a countermove, they often aren't ready for it. If you get an offensive lineman who jumps out there on a speed rush up the field, the next move you're going to try will often be a spin back inside. I did and Sharpe was right there.

That was a tribute to his mobility. If he had simply spent his off-season conditioning time in the weight room, he would not have been ready for my inside spin. But Sharpe studies the game. He works on his mobility, which you are doing every time you jump rope. And he stretches regularly to maintain his flexibility.

You should do the same. Don't think you are going to get by on strength alone.

WEEK 5

We have now completed what I consider a transitional period and are approaching our turning point.

Right now, you should be feeling pretty good about yourself. You have laid a good base for getting into football shape. You should be running a good pace on your half-mile and mile-and-a-half runs.

Now we're going to make a transition into more football-oriented exercises. We are going to specify our conditioning and eliminate some of the things that don't relate directly to football. For example, we will not be doing as much straight-ahead distance running. Now we want to get you accustomed to the type of movement that you will be doing on the football field. We will do that with the *shuttle drill*, which is a stop-and-go drill, where you run full speed in one direction, stop, then turn around and run full speed in the opposite direction.

No matter what position you play, you will probably have to do that numerous times throughout the course of a game. A perfect example would be when the Giants play the New Orleans Saints and I have to chase their fine running back, Dalton Hilliard. He might start a play running to his left, which is our defensive right. I will chase him over to that side. In an instant, he will see a hole and cut back in the other direction. It's an instinctive play for him. He runs, finds his route blocked, spots an opening, stops, cuts on a dime, and races through the hole on the other side.

While he's running around looking for daylight, it's my job to close the door on him. To be in on the play, I have to stop, change direction, and run full speed back to the hole that he is trying to get through. This is a reaction drill for defensive players. For offensive players, it is an action drill.

That's the purpose of doing the shuttle drill. It prepares you to make instant adjustments like the one needed to catch Hilliard on the play I just described. Football is a game of adjustments on the run. You have to change directions and get from Point A to Point B at full speed to get involved in a play and to make a tackle.

We will be focusing on football in other ways. For those of you who will be playing running back or wide receiver when the season opens, we will begin having you jog a mile while holding a football.

If you are a running back such as an Eric Dickerson and you are the primary focus of your team's rushing attack, you will probably carry the ball twenty to thirty times a game. You're going to take a lot of hits and you are going to have some long runs, which could tire you out.

When you jog a mile with a football in your hands, the first half-mile is going to be easy. You should think of that as being the first half of a football game.

But the final half-mile, like the second half of a football game, may not be so easy. The football may begin to feel awkward in your hands. You start to wish you weren't holding it, because it is hampering your running. Now is the time you really have to concentrate on making that football a part of your running, a part of your body. Think of it as running the football in the fourth period, when you're exhausted but the team needs one more first down. Because you're the workhorse of the offense, you have to get it for your team.

If you want to be able to do it then, you have to start doing it now. Jogging a mile with a football gets you used to running with the ball when you're tired, which is when you're most susceptible to fumbling. Concentration is the key. This is a mental, as well as a physical, exercise.

MONDAY

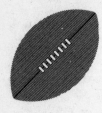

BREAKFAST: Start off with a glass of your preferred juice and half of a honeydew melon. Then we'll have a plate of pancakes and syrup or honey, plus a bagel or English muffin.

▼

LUNCH: Eat a bowl of chicken soup with rice or noodles and crackers. Our main course today will be a hot turkey sandwich on whole wheat bread, mashed potatoes, and carrots. Include a tossed salad with your meal. Drink water or juice with your lunch.

▼

DINNER: We'll try another fish dish tonight, broiled red snapper, one of my favorites. Our side dishes this evening will be rice and spinach. Don't drink soda with your dinner. For dessert, eat a banana or two.

Weigh yourself before working out, so you know how much fluid to drink when you weigh yourself after the workout is complete.

Warm up.

Stretch for 30 to 40 minutes.

Jump rope for 10 minutes. Do it in two 5-minute intervals if you like.

Run a half-mile at three-quarters the speed of your fastest half-mile. We are not running this half-mile for time. Its purpose is to warm your body and loosen the muscles for the work that lies ahead.

Walk a lap.

Run four 440s for time. Running a 440 may be the most difficult exercise that you do in this program. It is short enough to be considered a sprint, but not quite long enough to be a distance run. That makes it almost like a long-distance sprint.

It's not like running a half-mile or a mile. At those distances, you can pace yourself. But the 440 is run at a constant pace. You must go all out, because it is a difficult exercise.

But it's also a very good exercise for you, because it will help you become a strong runner by building up your stamina and en-

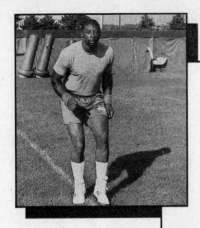

The 440-yard dash will build up both your stamina and your endurance.

When running sprints, do not slow down over the last 10 yards.

durance. These 440s will help you increase your endurance; they will train you to run faster for a longer period of time.

Jump rope for 10 minutes.

Warm down and stretch for 30 minutes.

Do your weight work.

Do 30 sit-ups and 30 push-ups.

Drink fluids to replace lost weight.

TUESDAY

BREAKFAST: Start with a glass of sugar-free juice and half a cantaloupe. Eat a healthful bowl or two of cold cereal, remembering to avoid sugar. As you should know by now, these include corn, bran, or wheat flakes or shredded wheat. Along with your cereal, eat an English muffin or toast with honey, our favorite natural sweetener.

LUNCH: Today we'll have baked chicken with mixed vegetables, as well as a tossed salad. If you want a somewhat lighter lunch, eat a chicken salad sandwich on the bread of your choice. Make sure to drink only healthful, fluid-replacement beverages. If you wish to have dessert, make it Jell-O, sherbet, or a piece of fruit.

▼

DINNER: We'll make this a big carbohydrates night and have spaghetti and meatballs for dinner. Have some green beans with that, as well as dinner rolls or bread. Drink water or juice with your meal. For dessert, eat a bowl of sherbet, low-fat frozen yogurt, or a banana.

Warm up.

Stretch for 30 to 40 minutes.

Jog a mile while holding a football. Concentrate on what you're doing and don't drop the ball. That's a fumble and you can't afford to do that in a game.

Do 15 minutes of football exercises and drills. As I said at the beginning of the week, we are beginning to focus on the football season with a greater sense of urgency. What follows are exercises that are specifically for football players. Some are tailored for certain positions. But that doesn't mean you should ignore those that don't pertain directly to your position.

Anything that improves your agility and awareness on the football field helps you become a better player. During the course of a game, you will have to perform many tasks. Several of them will certainly be out of the norm for your position and no one knows that better than me.

I demonstrated a perfect example of that during the fifth week of the 1989 season, when I caught a touchdown pass from Jeff Hostetler on a fake field goal during a game in Philadelphia against the Eagles. It was a classic example of why you should work on all your skills, not just the ones you think you're going to use regularly.

I am the wing man on the field goal team, on the end, just off the line of scrimmage. In practice, we have a lot of fun working on the fake. The tight end usually runs for the post and I run for the first down marker.

I never thought we would run it in a game. But on two previous field goals we had kicked, Andre Waters of the Eagles was rushing hard, whether or not the rush side of their defense was to his side. I went to the sideline and told Romeo Crennel, our special teams coach at the time, that they weren't checking for containment—they

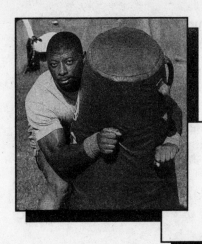

Practice all the football drills, even if they don't pertain specifically to your position.

weren't hesitating long enough to make sure we weren't running a fake. I told him I thought we could run the fake.

Normally, teams like to rush field goal attempts from the wide side of the field, the side opposite the hash mark on which the ball is placed. But there're usually one or two players who will tip you off as to which way the block is going. In Philadelphia, the key is Reggie White. Whichever side he's on, that's the side from which they're going to try and block the field goal.

Reggie White was lining up on the same side for every kick, so we figured they were concentrating their efforts there. Perhaps they thought we were weak on one side. I was the right wing. Reggie was lined up on the opposite side, our left side. Despite the rush side being over there, Andre Waters kept rushing from my side. He wasn't at all concerned with what I was doing.

After that happened two or three times, our head coach, Bill Parcells, asked me if I was ready to run the fake. I certainly was! I didn't think Hostetler was going to throw me the ball anyway, because in practice he always threw it to the tight end. But I knew I would be open and if he did toss it my way, I'd at least get the first down.

My job was to run a down-and-out to the first down marker. When the ball was snapped, Andre Waters rushed the kicker as he had done on the previous attempts. He ran right by me. I got to my assigned area, where I was open for about a month. Nobody was near me. Hostetler was still trying to find the tight end. Finally, he threw it to me. When it was in the air I was thinking, "This is my big chance."

I was concentrating so hard on the ball, it seemed like I saw every revolution it took. I wanted it to get to me before somebody realized I was wide open. The ball got there, I caught it, though I did bobble it a moment off my pads. I turned and headed for the goal line and scored. Touchdown. It was one of the most memorable plays of my career, because I was actually in on an offensive play.

Until that moment, all of the big plays in my career had come when I was lined up on defense, including my big touchdown in Atlanta in 1988. This was my first big offensive play and I came through when it counted.

After you've done that once, the coaches tell the quarterback to look for you the next two or three times you run that play. So I think I've given myself a chance to get more opportunities to make more touchdowns and first downs for the team.

Of course, it wasn't all perfect. After I scored the touchdown, we had to kick the extra point, which meant that the field goal team was supposed to stay on the field. Well, ten of them did. But after I went to the sideline to celebrate my touchdown, I forgot to go back out onto the field. Fortunately, Ottis Anderson was paying attention. He was my backup at the wing position on the kicking teams.

I made the big touchdown, but I forgot to take part in the extra point. That's something I'll have to concentrate on in the future.

I might never have made that big play if I had not taken the time during my workouts to practice catching a football. But the work I had put in during the off-season paid off on that play.

You don't have to do all of the following exercises in one day. Pick the ones you have the most trouble with and work hardest on those.

Focus on those exercises that pertain to your position, but don't ignore the others. You never know when you may be called on to do something else.

Here is a list of the drills you should do, in no particular order:

Line drills: Pick a yard line—start, for example, at the 20-yard line—and go to one sideline. Begin running at a 45-degree angle to the 25-yard line. When you reach the 25, cut back and, while moving at the same angle, run at another 45-degree angle back to the 20. Keep going in this manner until you reach midfield. Do this 4 times. Then increase your distance to 10 yards for a set of four, then 15

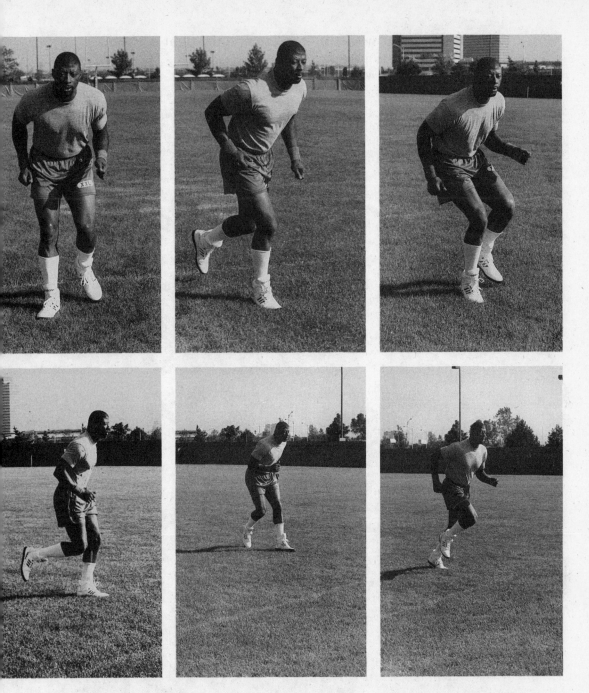

Line drills enable you to simulate running at an angle, an often overlooked but vital skill on the football field. As with all drills, you must concentrate fully and give a total effort from the first step to the last.

The swivel drill allows you to practice turning from side to side while backpedaling, which all linebackers and defensive backs must be able to do. In addition, the exercise will improve your agility and coordination while teaching you to keep your eye on the ball.

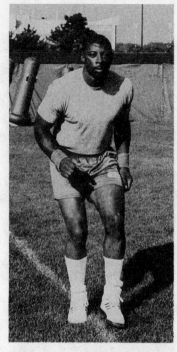

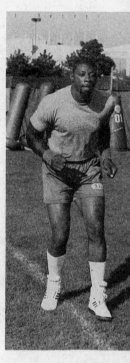

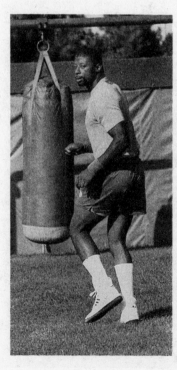

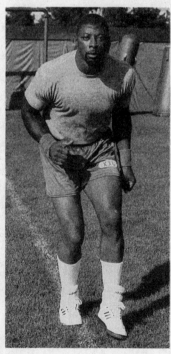

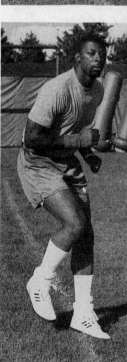

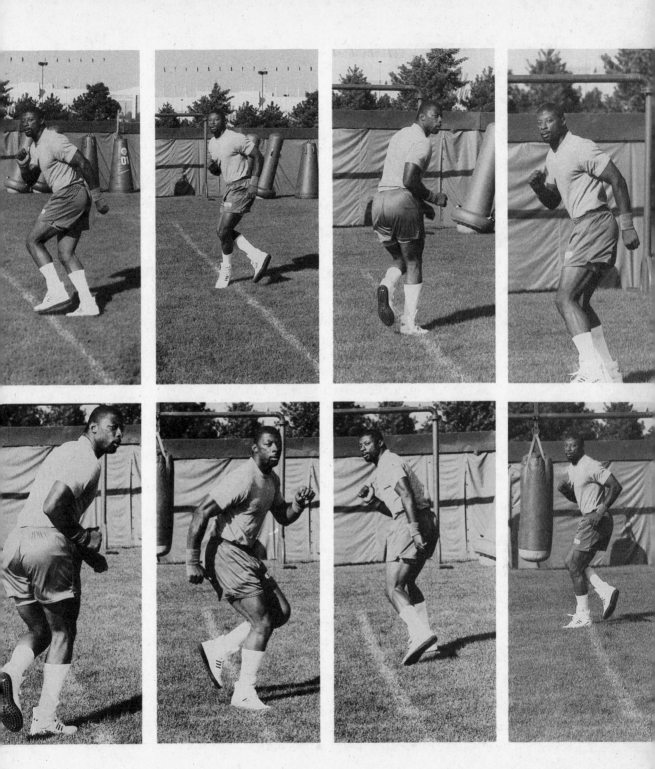

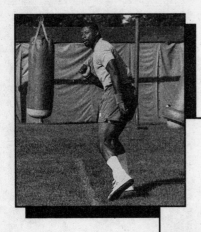

Shuttle drills and line drills will get you accustomed to the type of movement you do on a football field.

yards for another set of four. Remember, you are not running forward or backward. You are running at an angle.

If you are a linebacker and defensive back, line drills will get you feeling comfortable backing up as you watch a play develop, then breaking up toward the ball to make a tackle.

Swivel drill: Start on a yard line. While backpedaling, turn your hips and shoulders to one side while keeping your head facing straight ahead. Backpedal for 5 yards, then turn your body the opposite way while continuing to backpedal. Make sure to keep your head straight. Continue this way for 15 to 20 yards, then plant and sprint back to the original line.

Concentrate on backpedaling in a straight line. Work hard at not coming off that line.

Your head should always be looking the same way while backpedaling, while your shoulders and hips keep turning.

This drill improves your agility while disciplining you to keep your eye on the ball as you watch a play unfold.

Pass drops: This drill is exactly like it sounds. If you are a linebacker or defensive back, simulate dropping back as you would if you were covering a wide receiver or a running back running a pass pattern in a zone defense.

Drop back in a straight line and at several different angles. Once you've dropped back anywhere from 10 to 25 yards, pretend a pass has been thrown and sprint to the spot where the receiver would be.

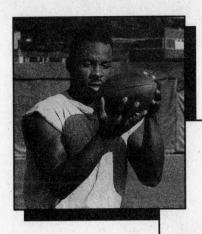

When you are catching a football, look the ball right into your hands.

Catching the ball: This is the advanced version of the pass drop. If you have a workout partner, take a pass drop and have him throw the ball to you. Your catch, of course, simulates an interception. Make sure to have your partner vary the angle of his throws. As a defensive player the ball will seldom be thrown right at you, because you're not the intended receiver. So have your partner throw it behind you, well in front of you, close to the ground, and high enough in the air for you to jump for it.

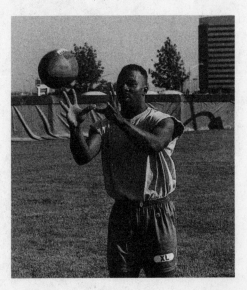

Always practice catching a football with your hands and not against your chest. Keep your fingers outstretched, catch the ball, and tuck it safely away.

Tire drills: If you can get about a dozen old tires, lay them out on the ground in two long rows. Then run through them with high steps. This will get you into the habit of picking your knees up when you run. It will also help improve your agility and balance.

Tackling a dummy: If you can, pick up a tackling dummy at your local sporting goods store or borrow one from your coach or school. Practice using proper tackling form, which includes keeping your head up, your eyes open, and wrapping your arms around the ballcarrier.

Sometimes you can't get a dummy, but you can get a person. Again, if you have an exercise partner, make use of him. If you are using a person, go through the approach full speed. Since you don't want to hurt your buddy, slow down before you make the tackle. Tackling form is more important than hitting your partner hard.

Practice your open field tackling. Have your partner start running toward you from 20 to 30 yards away. You can close the gap between the two of you, wait until the proper moment to commit, keep your eyes on his waist, and get into good tackling position. Again, your tackling form is more important than creaming your partner.

With a tackling dummy you can practice the three vital rules for tackling: Keep your head up, your eyes open, and wrap your arms around the ballcarrier.

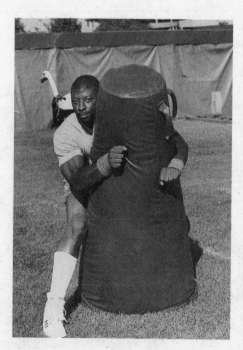
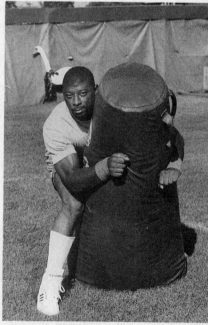

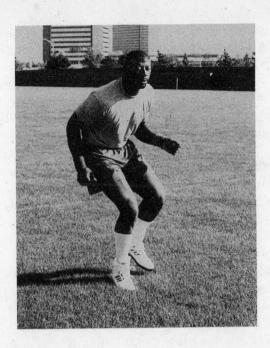

Backpedaling: This is a very basic, yet vital, skill for all line-backers and defensive backs. You will find yourself running backward in a variety of situations during the course of one play. Practice backpedaling, pick a spot on the field where you want to go, plant, and drive toward that spot. Also practice your stance and moving out of a stance.

Quarterback drills: Quarterbacks should take a lot of snaps from a center. Have someone hike you the ball. It may seem simple, but a lot of football games have been lost because of fumbled snaps. You can't execute a handoff or drop back to pass if you can't get the ball from your center.

Practice a variety of handoffs, including handing the ball off to the left and to the right. Many offenses now use pitchouts to get the ball outside to their backs quickly. Work on pitching the ball out to your left, then pitching it out to your right.

Get your throwing arm ready. Practice throwing the ball. Pick a stationary target and test your accuracy. If you have a workout partner, let him run pass patterns for you. Make sure you don't overthrow. The last thing a quarterback wants when he gets to training camp is a tired or sore arm.

Running back drills: Running backs should practice taking hand-offs and pitchouts from each side. On pitchouts, they should look the ball right into their hands. Make your first priority securing the ball in your hands. Don't start looking for holes to run through until you have the ball. If you don't, you won't have to worry about spotting holes, because you will be going back to pick up the ball you dropped.

A good drill for running backs is to have someone swipe at the ball when you're running with it. During games, unfriendly defenders will be trying all day to pry the ball loose from you. If you haven't prepared yourself, you could fumble it away.

In 1989, I set a team record by causing seven opposition fumbles, so I am well aware of how defensive players can victimize a ball-carrier who doesn't take care of the ball.

Backs should also high-step through tires while carrying the ball, as well as practice their different moves. Don't think you're going to get out on the field and make a defender look foolish with an unrehearsed head fake. You could get lucky and do that. But you will have a lot more confidence, as well as an extra trick or two, if you practice your fakes and moves.

Practice will help sharpen your instincts. At a given moment during a game, you may not be certain what fake you're going to use, but by practicing a variety of moves, you'll be able to pull a rabbit out of your hat when you need to.

Finally, offensive backs should practice catching forward passes, since they are increasingly asked to do this in modern football.

Wide receiver drills: Wide receivers should, of course, practice catching the ball. Have someone throw you many different kinds of passes, including short, medium, and long tosses. Get used to catching the ball with your hands instead of trapping it with your body. Look the ball all the way into your hands and then tuck it under your arm. You should do it all in one motion, so that protecting the ball becomes second nature to you.

Practice catching the ball over each shoulder, while leaping off the ground with your arms stretched high above your head, as well as diving for balls thrown low near the ground. If the ground is hard, use some padding to land on while practicing. A game situation is different. That's when you have to make that extra effort for the ball, so a few grass stains will be worth it.

Footwork is also critical to wide receivers. Unless you have blinding speed, you are going to have to rely on your moves to get open. That requires fancy feet. Do a lot of agility drills to develop quick feet. Jumping rope is excellent.

Practice catching the ball near each sideline and coming down in bounds. Do the same thing at the back of the end zone and with an imaginary first down marker.

Another skill important to wide receivers is releasing off the line of scrimmage. Have your partner call out a snap count and practice coming off the line as quickly as you can. Then try to do it with someone jamming you, which is what you will face during the course of a game. This is where footwork is most important, as well as those instinctive fakes you'll be practicing.

As a receiver you won't be called on to block very often and when you do it will largely be just getting in a defender's way. We call that *stalk blocking*. You are occupying a defender, standing in his way. You can practice stalk blocking with your partner.

Linemen drills: Yes, you need a lot of strength to be successful up front. But you can't get by on strength alone. You also need agility, no matter which side of the ball you are on. Both offensive and defensive linemen should do a lot of footwork exercises. This is where jumping rope should pay off for you bigger guys.

Offensive linemen should simulate both run and pass blocking. Get in your stance and practice firing out to block for a running play. Return to your stance and practice getting back in pass protection position.

Defensive linemen should work on coming quickly out of their stance, because the first step or two are critical for rushing linemen. They should simulate going up against a guard or tackle. Defensive linemen should also practice pursuing the ball.

Hand speed is very important. Get a hand-held pad, which we call a *shiver pad*, and work on getting your hands up quickly and hitting a blocker.

Defensive back drills: Defensive backs can never do too many footwork drills. A cornerback or safety should put a lot of emphasis on developing good, quick feet. Backpedal, side-to-side, and hip swivel drills all help the players in the secondary develop the skills they absolutely must have to succeed.

If you play in the secondary, you should practice catching the ball, just as if you were a receiver.

If you are a wide receiver or a running back, you should practice catching as many balls as you can. They should be thrown long-, short-, and medium-range, high and low, and in front of you and behind you. Be careful to catch the ball with your hands, not your body.

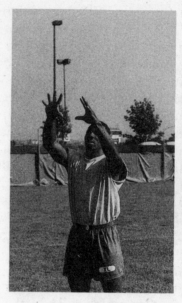
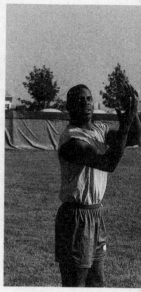
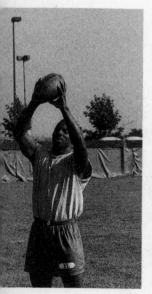
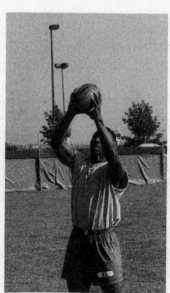
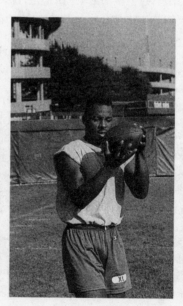
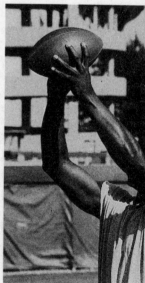

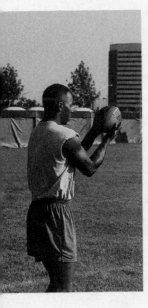 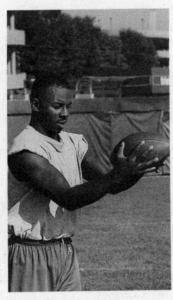 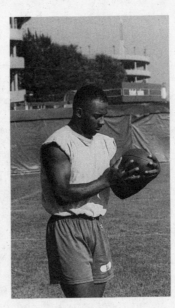 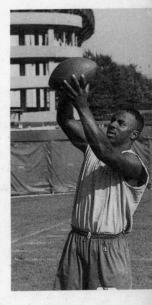

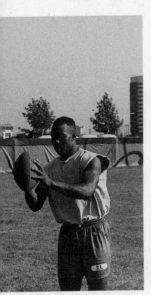 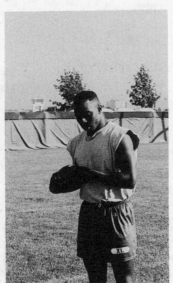 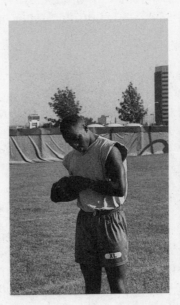 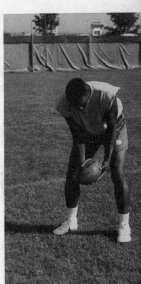

Work on covering receivers man-to-man. Also, practice your tackling, particularly open-field tackling, because that's where most tackles by defensive backs are going to come. And in many cases, you will be the last line of defense.

WEDNESDAY

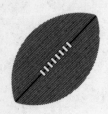

BREAKFAST: Start off with a glass of your favorite juice. Continue with a grapefruit half, then have French toast with syrup or honey. If that doesn't provide enough fuel for your workout day, eat a piece or two of fruit or an English muffin.

▼

LUNCH: Let's have a bowl of beef noodle soup with crackers, followed by baked macaroni and cheese. If you prefer eating sandwiches, make it turkey, chicken, or tuna fish on whole wheat bread. Don't forget to include a salad and your fluid-replacement beverages.

▼

DINNER: Tonight, we'll have baked fillet of sole. Fill out the meal with some green beans or peas, rice and rolls, bread or cornbread. For dessert, eat green or red grapes.

Weigh yourself before working out.
Warm up.
Stretch for 30 to 40 minutes.
Run a half-mile at three-quarter speed.

Now we're going to start doing shuttle runs, in this case a 200-yard shuttle run. That means you sprint 50 yards, run back 50 yards to your starting point, sprint for 50 more yards, then turn and run back again. A shuttle run has no rest stops. You have to turn and keep going.

You might wonder why you shouldn't just run 200 yards in one clip. A shuttle run lets you go the same distance, but it is a much more football-oriented drill. If possible, do your shuttle runs on a grass field or some other type of football playing surface. And do them carrying a football if you are a running back, wide receiver, or defensive back. If you are going to do a drill that is so closely tied with the sport, it makes sense to do everything you can to simulate a game condition.

Do four 200-yard shuttle runs. You will probably be a bit tired toward the end of your shuttle runs, but keep running as hard as you can. And make sure you don't drop the football.

Make sure you drink plenty of fluids.

When you are finished with your shuttle runs, jog a half-mile with the ball. This will allow you to warm down.

Stretch for 30 minutes.

Do your football drills. At this point in the program, I believe it is wise to do as many drills as possible, no matter what position you play. Even if you are an offensive lineman, it can't hurt you if you do some of the defensive back drills. As my fake field goal touchdown in Philadelphia proved, you never know when you'll be called on to use an unfamiliar skill.

Later on in the program, as we get closer to training camp, you can concentrate on the drills that pertain to your position.

Do your weight work.

Finish with 30 sit-ups and 30 push-ups.

THURSDAY

BREAKFAST: Begin the day with a glass of juice, then pineapple rings or a cantaloupe half. Continue with a plain omelet and some pancakes (plain or apple) or English muffins. Make sure to eat some honey today.

▼

LUNCH: Chicken soup with rice or noodles, then eat one or two hamburgers. Take care to see that they are made with very lean ground beef. If you prefer cheeseburgers, use only low-fat cheese. You should eat these hamburgers at home. Don't go to a fast-food restaurant. With your burgers, eat wax beans and a mixed green salad. Don't forget to drink plenty of fluid-replacement beverages.

▼

DINNER: Let's stick with fish and eat baked cod. Be sure to avoid tartar sauce and flavor it instead with lemon. Complement that with a side dish of spaghetti, as well as peas and cauliflower and dinner rolls. For dessert, eat a banana, orange, or pear.

> Warm up.
> Stretch for 30 to 40 minutes.
> Jump rope for 15 minutes. You can do it all at once or break it up into three 5- or two 7½-minute intervals.
> Jog a half-mile carrying a football.
> Do football exercises for 15 to 30 minutes.
> Stretch for 15 minutes.
> Do 30 sit-ups and 30 push-ups.

I understand at this point that the program may seem a little repetitious. Each year at about this point in the program, I get a desire to spend my time at other pursuits. It is more than a month since we started working and the football season seems like it is far away.

But to slack off now would defeat the whole purpose of starting the program in the first place. You would be taking conditioning for granted, figuring you have done enough to coast the rest of the way. But if I have learned anything in my football career it is never, ever take anything for granted.

John Elway is a player who has demonstrated to me why it's important to never take anything for granted on a football field.

He has an excellent sense on the field that helps him avoid a pass rush. Elway is very good at deciphering a defense. He knows how to throw on the run. If he is scrambling one way, he can turn and throw the ball clear across the field for a 50-yard touchdown.

When we played the Broncos in Super Bowl XXI, I had a blind side shot at him and he got away. He didn't see me coming. But at the last second, something told him to look. Instead of me sacking him for a loss, Elway ran the ball and gained a few yards.

I will never again assume I have John Elway trapped until I see him on the ground.

FRIDAY

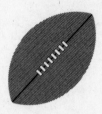

BREAKFAST: Start your day with a glass of juice, plus a grapefruit half or pear. Then have a bowl of cold cereal, taking care to avoid those that have been pre-sugared. Finish up with French toast and sugar or, for a bit lighter fare, toast and honey.

▼

LUNCH: A bowl of vegetable soup with crackers to start with. Because I'm not sure if you'll be getting your carbohydrates over the weekend, eat a plate of fettucine or spaghetti with tomato or red clam sauce. If you would rather not eat that much, stick with our traditional turkey sandwich on whole wheat bread. Eat carrots with either entrée and don't forget a salad and healthful beverages.

▼

DINNER: It's Friday, so you can have a treat. Tonight enjoy a lean sirloin steak. Be sure to trim away all the excess fat. With your steak, have mushrooms, broccoli, and a baked potato, plus dinner rolls and bread. For dessert, have a bowl of ice milk or low-fat frozen yogurt with strawberries.

Weigh yourself before working out.

Warm up.

Stretch for 30 to 40 minutes.

Jump rope for 10 minutes.

Run a fast-paced half-mile for time. Try to improve on your last timed half-mile and make sure you aren't slowing down.

Run three 440s for time, walking a lap in between and after the last one.

Stretch for another 15 to 20 minutes to get your body ready for the shorter sprints you are about to run.

Replenish your fluids.

Now run two 300-yard shuttles. They are, of course, very similar to the 200-yard shuttles you ran on Wednesday except now you have to sprint an extra 50 yards in each direction. And don't forget to carry that football if you're a running back, receiver, or defensive back. Make sure you don't drop it!

Walk a lap and stretch.

Do at least 15 minutes of football drills.

Do your weight work.

Finish the day with 30 push-ups and 30 sit-ups.

THE WEEKEND

Warm up, stretch, and soak.

After three weeks of weight lifting, you may not be satisfied with the amount of weight you've added, if gaining weight is indeed your goal. Because of that, you may think you have to eat a lot more food to reach your weight goals.

But Ronnie Barnes has taught me that to gain one to two extra pounds of muscle a week, you need to take in an additional 700 to 1,000 healthful calories per day. That will fuel the weight training you're doing and provide the extra calories you need for your tissue. That's a lot of extra calories. Where can you fit them in? The easiest way to get them is to stick to the balanced diet we've stressed since day one of this program.

If you still believe you're not getting all you need, add some extra skim milk, extra fruit juice, and a low-fat liquid meal to your diet. If you use skim milk, you will get extra protein and carbohydrates without extra fat.

Another point I want to emphasize again is that you must get enough rest to excel in this program. The more motivated you are, the less you might consider the importance of proper rest.

A good night's sleep enables your muscles to recover and store your energy reserves so you can work to full capacity each day. Make sure you are getting enough sleep. If you are feeling fatigued because of the demands of the program, take a nap during the day. But don't deny yourself the rest you need.

WEEK 6

We are now beginning the second half of the program. You should be thinking more and more about the coming football season, which is just around the corner. The work you do now is the beginning of a successful season. Everything you do now is directly related to football.

You should be thinking about the football season when you're getting tired and you don't feel like going all out or completing everything you set out to do. But if you cheat yourself now, you'll be cheating yourself in the game. You should be thinking, "I may not be able to break that long run when I need it if I don't make the effort to get in shape now."

As a football player, you can never tell when that situation is going to come up. It's something you can't dictate, so you have to condition your body for whenever it does happen.

If you talk to any good running back, he will tell you that he wants every run to be a big run. That's the kind of positive attitude you need to have. Of course, every run is not going to be a long touchdown. But if and when you do break a long one, your body has to be able to respond to it.

The same rules apply if you're a defensive player. As a linebacker, I say to myself, "What if I'm in a footrace with a tight end like Steve Jordan of the Minnesota Vikings or Robert Awalt of the Phoenix Cardinals?" Will I be able to catch him. They're very crafty guys who are very capable of getting a step on me. If I'm in a footrace with either one of them, they're going to want to win it and so am I.

Am I going to be in condition to take away what he wants or is he going to be in better condition and obtain his goal?

I know that if I want to enjoy a favorable outcome to that dilemma, I have to put in a solid effort every day during my off-season workout.

MONDAY

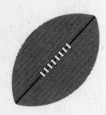

BREAKFAST: Begin your day with a glass of juice. Today we'll have a fruit cocktail, an English muffin with honey, and French toast with syrup.

▼

LUNCH: We'll continue to eat a lot of soup, because it's good energy food. Today, we'll have a bowl of pea soup with crackers. When you've finished that, eat chicken, preferably baked, with broccoli. Don't forget the green salad. Drink fluid-replacement beverages.

▼

DINNER: For our main course tonight, we'll try a cornish hen with stuffing, green beans, corn, and dinner rolls (without butter), plus our usual healthful beverages. A banana or peaches will make a nice dessert.

Weigh yourself before departing for your workout.
Warm up.
Stretch for 30 to 40 minutes. If you have kept up all the way, you have been stretching at least six days a week for five weeks. Your hamstrings, groin, and quadriceps feel good and loose, and on many of the leg stretches you can get your head down further than you ever thought you could. If you are like some players, you may think you don't have to stretch as much before and after every workout. You may think it would be wiser to use the time doing something else, like shuttle runs or bench presses.

I can state flatly that such thinking is wrong. It is very important that you keep stretching every day for at least the 30 or 40 minutes you have been doing it to this point. In December, when the NFL season is winding down, I spend just as much if not more time stretching than I do when training camp opens in July. You should never shortchange yourself when it comes to stretching.

If you don't stretch thoroughly, you run a great risk of pulling a muscle and forcing yourself to the sidelines for at least 30 days. You never wake up in the morning with your body totally stretched. And you can't take it for granted that your muscles are going to stretch by themselves. There is no such thing as being naturally stretched or naturally flexible. Your muscles work, they get tired, and you have to keep stretching them. You can always do a little bit more to stretch your muscles and warm them up.

At this stage it's very, very important that you continue to stretch. You're getting close to the season and you don't want to go to practice with a pulled muscle. It only slows you down and puts you behind everyone else. In a lot of systems there is no time for catch-up, so you're behind for the entire year.

After stretching, jump rope for 10 to 15 minutes.

Do four 330-yard shuttle runs. Go all out. Walk a lap in between the running.

Drink fluids as needed.

Warm down and stretch.

Do 15 minutes of football work. This can be anything football-related that requires agility, including catching passes, running pass patterns, and, if you're a linebacker or defensive back, taking pass drops.

Stretch briefly.

Do your weight work, including 25 sit-ups and 25 push-ups.

Don't forget to weigh yourself when you get home, and replace any fluids you have lost.

TUESDAY

BREAKFAST: Begin the day with your glass of juice and some pineapple rings or cantaloupe. Continue with a plain omelet with ham slices (make sure you trim any fat) and an English muffin, toast, or bagel. Make sure to eat some honey.

▼

LUNCH: Let's have some pizza today, since we all like it. Feel free to include your favorite topping, but make sure to go easy if it's pepperoni or sausage—that stuff's tasty, but it's not very good for you. I prefer peppers and mushrooms. Make sure you eat a tossed salad with that and drink plenty of fluid-replacement beverages. Stay away from soda.

▼

DINNER: Tonight, we'll enjoy some baked fillet of sole or baked flounder. Fill out the meal with some green beans, peas, rice, and cornbread or rolls. For dessert, try a piece of fruit pie, such as cherry, apple, or blueberry.

Warm up.

Stretch for 30 to 40 minutes.

Run a half-mile for time, making sure that you are at least keeping the same pace you established earlier.

Stretch for 10 to 15 minutes to prepare for shorter sprint work.

Do ten 110-yard dashes at three-quarter speed. *Be careful not to slow down over the last 10 or 20 yards.*

This last point is very important. When you run sprints in a noncompetitive environment, there is often a tendency to slow down over the last several yards. That might not hurt you if nothing is at stake. But it can be costly on a football field.

If you get in the habit of going all out now, it will carry over to the times when you are wearing a uniform. Running a complete 110-yard dash now helps put your running into a football framework.

In a game, you may be trying to catch a guy who is trying to run 80 yards for a touchdown. If you're used to conking out after 70 yards, you can never make up that step. But if you are accustomed to going 100 yards full speed, then you have an advantage, because you know you can run at your top speed for as long as the ball-carrier can possibly go. But if you are conditioning your body to go a shorter distance and then slow down, that is what is going to naturally happen if you're in that situation during a game. The man you're chasing will beat you every time.

You have to be a strong finisher, no matter what position you play. If you are a running back or a wide receiver and you're going to break a long run or catch a touchdown bomb, and you have conditioned yourself to slow up before completing your task, there's a good chance that you'll get caught from behind.

So go all out for the full distance. It will give you a big edge on the football field.

After you've finished running, warm down and stretch again.

Do 15 minutes of football-related agility exercises.

Stretch. The reason you are stretching so often today is that you are doing a lot of different exercises at a lot of different distances. You can't take for granted that being stretched out for a half-mile means you are stretched out properly to run 110-yard dashes. It's important to continually stretch, because the distances change and each distance taxes different muscles. Stretching once will not prepare you for a full day of workouts. Never think that one stretch will satisfy you for the entire day.

Don't forget to drink replacement fluids regularly.

WEDNESDAY

BREAKFAST: Begin the day with a glass of juice, followed by a honeydew melon or pear halves. Then have a bowl or two of healthful hot cereal, plus toast with honey.

▼

LUNCH: Let's begin with chicken soup with noodles or rice. Move on to lasagna with a side dish of green beans. Include a mixed green salad. When you eat your daily lunch salad, I hope you are remembering to stay away from dressings that are heavy in fat, such as Thousand Island or blue cheese. Stick to low-fat dressings. Drink water or juice with your meal and have fruit for dessert.

▼

DINNER: Tonight we'll have roast pork loin with applesauce. Have mixed vegetables with that, as well as a baked potato and dinner rolls or bread. Remember, use little or no butter on either. Treat yourself to an ice milk dessert.

Weigh yourself before working out.

Warm up.

Stretch for 30 to 40 minutes.

Jump rope for 10 minutes.

Do six 220-yard dashes. Make sure you run for the full distance on every one. Walk a lap in between each.

Warm down and stretch.

Do 15 minutes of football-agility drills. This is the point of the program where I really begin to focus on my specific duties on the football field. One of those is defending the pass. I begin practicing my pass drops, running backward then rushing forward or back toward the ball, as I would when covering a pass during a game.

When you pass in an unsupervised game of touch football on your neighborhood field, pass coverage involves nothing more than picking out a man and trying to stay close enough to him so he doesn't catch a pass. In organized football, it's a bit more complicated. But the ultimate purpose is the same: Don't let the offensive team complete a pass.

Defensive football teams on the elementary, high school, collegiate, and professional levels use two basic types of defenses to try and stop an offensive passing attack. They are, simply enough, a zone defense and a man-to-man defense.

A *zone defense* is an area defense. It is designed to keep everything in front of you in a confined area. When you are playing a zone defense, you are really determining what area you want the offensive team to throw the ball to, as well as what you're going to give up. In the defense that I play in with the Giants, that is basically a pass that's 2 to 5 yards beyond the line of scrimmage. That's the only area that we don't cover, that we're not held responsible for in a zone. A 2-yard pass will rarely hurt you, so it doesn't make sense to use energy and players to defend it.

I've been playing zone defenses since my earliest days in football. Even on the Daily Tigers, Coach Haywood designed all of our pass defenses to be zones. Man-to-man defenses were very complicated at that level, plus the offenses were very creative, which made it harder to shut them down with man-to-man defenses.

A zone is a safe and somewhat conservative defense. Zone defenses are most effective when the offensive team is in its own territory, more than 50 yards from the goal line. When it is that far away from the goal line, the defense has more room to work. The

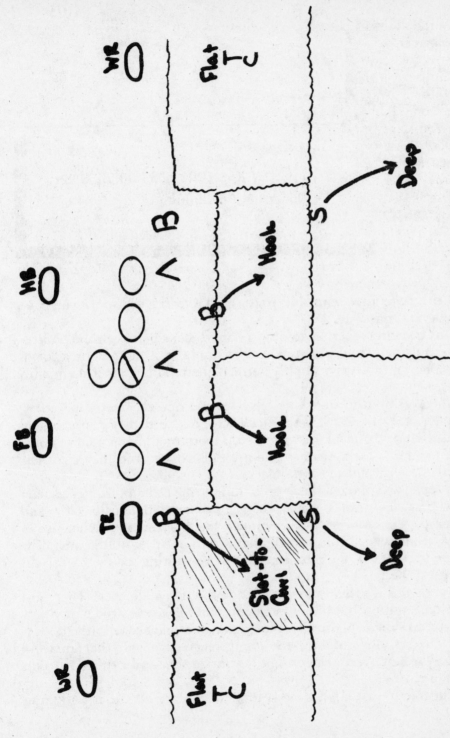

These are the areas a defense has to cover when it is defending a passing attack with a zone defense. The safeties are responsible for the two deep areas. The cornerbacks have the areas in the flat, closer to the sideline. Inside linebackers cover the hook area behind the line of scrimmage. As an outside linebacker, I am often responsible for the slot-to-curl area behind and to the side of the linemen.

133

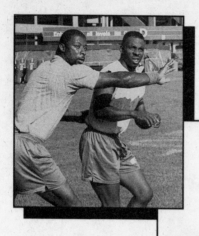

The key to a zone pass defense is individual discipline.

closer an offensive team gets to the goal line, the less space you have to operate in a zone.

Our decision whether to play a zone is based on both the opposition and their field position. For example, if a team runs a lot of crossing routes, it is probably better to match up against them with a zone.

The Washington Redskins have several fine receivers, including Art Monk, Gary Clark, and Ricky Sanders, and they run crossing routes all day. The Giants try to stop them by playing a lot of zone. The Phoenix Cardinals also run a lot of crosses, and they use their tight end with the wide receivers.

A zone is good if you have prepared for the crossing routes as part of your game plan, because then you know what to look for and when they're coming. It's very much like playing a zone defense in basketball, where you pass the man from one area to the next. The defender that's in the next area has to be waiting for the ball to get there.

There are disadvantages to playing a zone defense. The most obvious, and probably the most common, is getting too many people in one area. Naturally, that's going to leave you with too few defenders trying to cover too many receivers in another area. An observant quarterback is going to notice this and exploit it to his advantage.

The key to playing a zone is to be disciplined. You have to know what area you're willing to give up, while holding firm in the area that you want to defend. If I am covering the tight end 12 yards from the line of scrimmage and I see a running back standing alone 7 yards in front of me, I can't leave the tight end to go get the running back. That would be playing right into the hands of the quarterback, who would then complete a pass for a longer gain to the tight end I just left. If he does throw to the running back, then I break from my receiver to go up and make the tackle. That 5-yard completion is not going to hurt us as much as the 12-yarder would have.

In many of the defenses on the Giants, I have responsibility in what we call the *slot-to-curl area*, which is an area not more than 15 yards from the line of scrimmage, between the yard line numbers on the field and the hash marks (see diagram). As soon as I see the offense is going to throw a pass, I have to drop back into my area. Anything that comes into that slot area or that curl area is mine.

But I only carry the receiver so far. If somebody is streaking down the field and he comes through my area, I have to try and reroute that individual toward one of my defensive teammates, instead of toward the open area he hopes to find. I must change his pattern so that he's no longer running a direct route. Most of the time, that's with body position; I make him take an arc around me.

An important thing to remember in a zone is that I can't follow the receiver too far out of my area. If I follow him, it is almost certain that another receiver will also follow him into my area on a crossing pattern. So my job is to reroute the receiver, make sure he's been released to the next guy, such as a safety, and watch for somebody else coming into my area.

Sometimes you have to follow the receiver out of your area for a step or two. You have to make sure he doesn't stop as soon as he gets past you, because then he can hook up right there and catch a pass. Teams often try to spread the zone out, then hit a receiver underneath.

Whenever you play in a zone defense, make sure you see the quarterback. He is the guy throwing the ball. In a zone, it's very difficult to prevent a receiver from catching a pass if you can't see where that pass is coming from.

When we carry a receiver through our area to the next defender, we say we are using our *escort service*. It doesn't literally mean walking him over and saying, "You got him," but you have to take

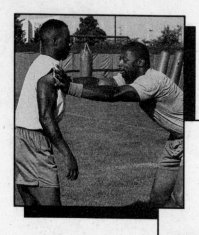

Don't look at the receiver when you are covering him in a man-to-man defense.

him to a point where you know the next defender can get to him. Without this kind of teamwork and accountability, a zone defense quickly and completely breaks down.

The other basic pass defense is, of course, the *man-to-man*. In that defense, you want to try and match up your best defenders against the opposition's finest receivers. When a team has a great quarterback, a man-to-man is often the best defense to be in. If he is facing a zone and has a lot of time to pass, then he can pick that zone apart, no matter how proficient your escort service is.

With a man-to-man, you know that one of three things is going to happen. You are going to cover all the receivers and the defensive linemen will sack the quarterback. Or the quarterback will have time to pass, but his receivers will be covered. The third possibility is not as beneficial to the defense. That is, of course, when one or more receivers are open and the quarterback has time to pass. The result is the dreaded completed pass.

In most man-to-man defenses on the Giants, I have a defensive teammate somewhere on the field who will give me help. It is usually a safety, who often has his eye on the other team's most dangerous receiver. As a man-to-man defender, it is very important to know where your help is. If you're playing man-to-man defense, you most often want to force the receiver to go inside, which is where the help will be. No one is a great man-to-man pass defender forever. You may be the best defender in the world, but if the quarterback has time, and the receiver has time, they'll find a way

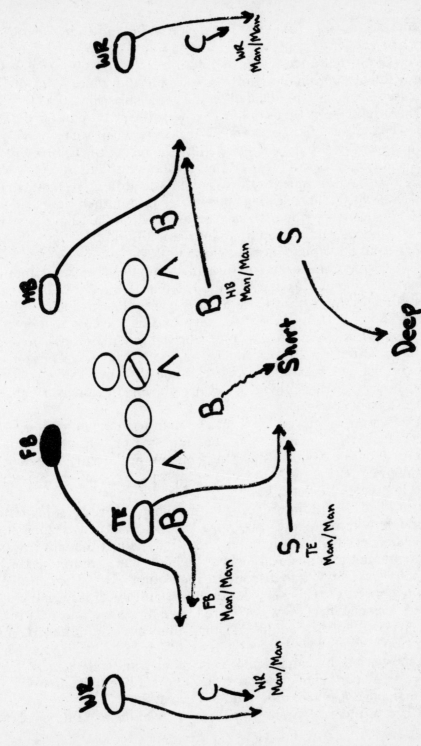

The responsibilities change when the defense is playing a man-to-man. Instead of covering an area, the defender is guarding a receiver. In this scheme, the cornerbacks are responsible for covering the two wide receivers. The strong safety has the tight end, while the strong-side outside linebacker, which for the Giants is usually me, watches the back coming out of the backfield. The free safety provides help should one of the receivers run a deep route.

to complete a pass. You have to use your help and count on a good pass rush.

The Giants are a team that likes to mix up its pass coverages. We use a lot of combinations of man-to-man and zone. A lot of the defenses we use are predicated on the game situation.

There have been times when I've been the only man on the defense in man-to-man coverage. That occurs when we're playing a team that passes to the tight end a lot. The rest of the Giants will be in a zone defense and I'll play man-to-man on the tight end. We've done that, for example, against the Philadelphia Eagles and Keith Jackson, who is an excellent pass receiver. Another tight end we need to cover that way is Ozzie Newsome of the Cleveland Browns. He is too good and too smart to let roam around in a zone: Bernie Kosar would complete passes to him all day.

My proudest achievement in a man-to-man coverage situation occurred when I was playing man-to-man while my teammates were functioning primarily in a zone. It was the third game of our Super Bowl season, 1986. We were in Los Angeles to play the Raiders, whose tight end was Todd Christensen, then considered the best pass-catcher at his position in the league. That day, Christensen caught just four passes for 27 yards. None of them occurred when I was directly responsible for guarding him. It was a performance I am still very proud of.

The reason we played the tight end man-to-man while the rest of the defense was in a zone is that Christensen was the primary offensive target. My task was a very big one at the time. I've done it many times in practice, but Christensen was very crafty, almost like another wide receiver.

But I had a lot of things going for me when I played against him. I could jam him in any direction, knowing there was zone help anywhere on the field. He never knew that; he just thought it was a straight man-to-man coverage. For the most part, I didn't need a lot of help. The plan was to discourage their quarterback, Jim Plunkett, from going to Christensen. He couldn't wait forever for Christensen to get open. When he was covered, he had to try and find other receivers. Plunkett couldn't do that often enough and the Giants won a big game, 14–9.

Christensen did catch some passes that game, but none of them were significant enough to hurt the Giants. I like to think my man-to-man coverage had a lot to do with that.

Once you learn how to play it, pass coverage should be a lot of

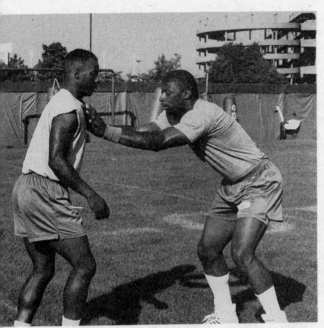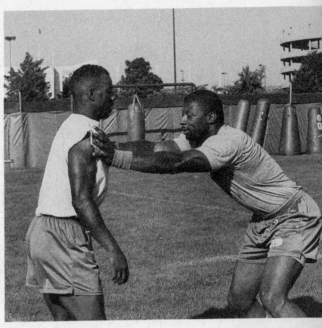

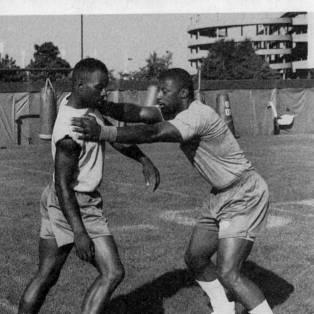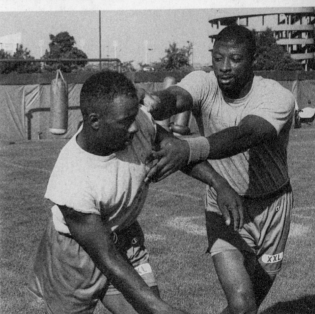

Jamming a wide receiver is a very effective technique for a defender. It delays the receiver, it forces him to fight just to get off the line of scrimmage, and it often makes him veer from his intended route.

fun. In the Giants' system, pass defense is very difficult to learn. Coming from the colleges to pro football, you learn that there is a lot more to a zone defense than just the area you're playing. You have to know different pass routes, including what route complements another route. There's so much you have to recognize. It's not just a matter of dropping back into an area and breaking toward the ball.

You have to know exactly what the offensive team is doing. If you don't, and they're successful running a particular play against you, they will keep doing it.

When you are covering a receiver in a man-to-man defense, chances are that your body will be between the receiver and the quarterback. Then you would use what we call the *trail technique*. You must keep your eyes focused on the receiver's waist, which is the most stable part of his body. Then you get close behind him and trail him until the play is over. Use the trail technique when you are covering the guys underneath. That places you between the receiver and the quarterback.

In a man-to-man, you can't look at the quarterback. The receiver is your responsibility, so you have to keep your eyes on him. You can't even sneak a peak at the quarterback until the receiver has declared his pattern or his pattern is completed. If you take a peak, you're beat.

One of the keys to playing man-to-man, which I haven't quite mastered yet, is patience. Knowing your receiver. Knowing the down and distance and being aware of where the offensive team has to go for a first down.

It all ties in together. For example, if you are covering a tight end, and he runs farther than 10 to 15 yards without making any kind of move or fake, then you have an 85 percent chance that he's going to run some kind of deep route. If he starts making moves anywhere up to 10 yards, then you must have an idea what he's going to do, what his favorite move is and how to counter it.

Although I am proud of the success I've had covering many of the NFL's best tight ends, one of my weaknesses still is covering a running back who has great moves. Trying to stay with a Stump Mitchell all afternoon was never my idea of fun.

The most difficult time I ever had covering a back was in practice early in my career, when I had to guard Tony Galbreath, who is now retired. I dreaded practicing against Tony. But doing it day in and

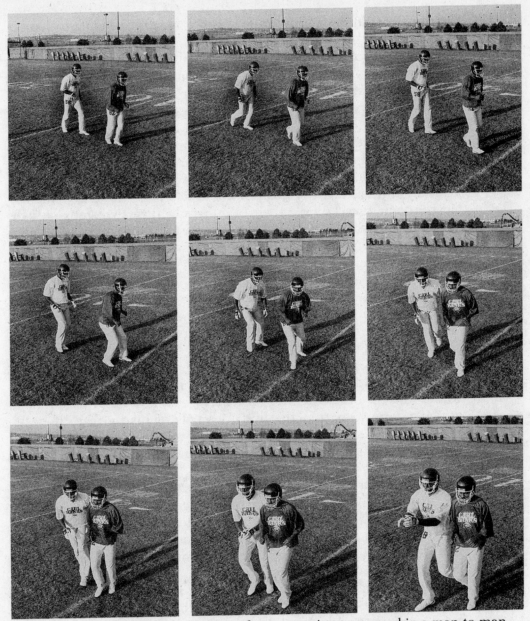

You must excel at the trail technique if you are going to succeed in a man-to-man defense. When using this technique, you follow, or trail, the receiver you are covering. It enables you to stay between the quarterback, who has the ball, and the receiver, who wants the ball. If you can't trail him closely enough, he's going to get it.

day out taught me a great deal about how to play a man-to-man defense.

While covering Tony, I learned that it is important for me to understand my position at all times. Tony was great at reading a defender and making him declare right away what position that defender was going to take on him. If we were practicing and I took an inside position, that meant I didn't want him to go inside. If I took an outside position, I would be trying to keep him from going toward the sideline.

But Tony was a master of deception. He would come out of the backfield and render my positioning useless. He would give me the best outside fake I'd ever seen. Tony would take two steps outside and look back as if he was searching for the ball and then turn around and come back inside on me. If I wasn't telling myself over and over again to take the inside away, I would bite on his outside fake.

It took great discipline not to go for the fake. I learned not to fall for it by knowing exactly what I wanted to do and sticking to it. The lessons that Tony Galbreath taught me in 1984, '85, and '86 are still important to me on the field today.

You won't be able to scout your opponents like we can in the NFL. But you should be aware of downs and distance. You should also know who the other team's best receiver is and watch to see if he is making a move within the first 10 yards of his pattern. If he is, you're going to have to close your trail technique down. You should start out about 3 feet behind the guy, but if he makes a move, you have to close it down a notch.

Football is a physical game, but knowledge of yourself and the opposition can help give you an advantage.

If you are a defensive back or a linebacker, chances are that you are going to have opportunities to intercept a pass. You can make the most of them by using your head and following a few simple rules.

First, look the ball all the way into your hands, just as a receiver is supposed to do when he is about to catch a pass. In that situation, you become the receiver. If you know you are about to get an interception, and you look upfield too early in your search for open running room, you are going to drop the ball. Any receiver will tell you you have to look the ball all the way into your hands before you do anything else. The premise is the same for what your baseball coach tells you when you go up to hit: Keep your eyes on the ball.

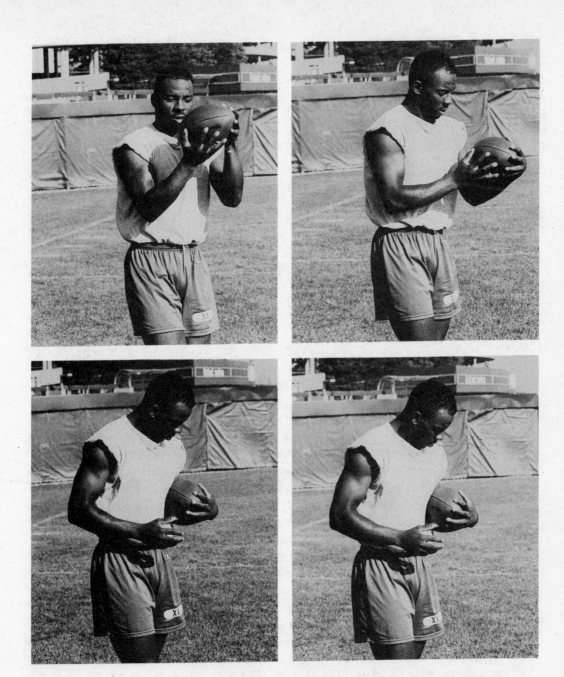

As soon as you catch a forward pass, tuck the ball under your arm and hold it tight, just as a running back does after taking a handoff or pitchout. This will greatly reduce your chances of fumbling, because it is very difficult for an opposing player to knock the ball away from you if it is secure under your arm.

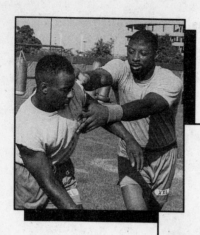

Tackling is an important skill for any football player.

On the Giants, the defensive players prepare for interceptions by doing many of the same drills the wide receivers do. One that I pay particular attention to is getting my hands in the proper position to catch the ball. I try to put my thumbs and forefingers together to form a diamond so the ball can fit right into my hands.

That technique is best used when you know the ball is coming right at you. On an interception, however, the quarterback is not trying to throw the ball to you. You have to take the attitude that the ball may be headed toward somebody else, but it's yours.

Rule number one is to catch the ball. Rule number two is to tuck it away. Only after you have followed the first two rules can you begin to run upfield. But make sure you don't take too long to do numbers one and two, or there will be no number three.

Sometimes a defensive player has to quickly change roles and become a blocker. That happens when a defender intercepts a pass or scoops up a fumble. The defensive team immediately takes on an offensive mind-set and tries to advance the ball. I've had the good fortune to actually intercept a pass, but my task on a turnover usually is as a blocker.

If you intercept a pass, don't take off on a haphazard run up the field. In that situation, think of yourself as a running back. Know where your blockers are and use them.

The most important principle to remember on interceptions is that the guy with the ball should try to get to the nearest hash mark. That means he doesn't have to go all the way across the field to find his blockers. If you get to the nearest hash mark, your blockers will find you.

If a defensive back or linebacker has the ball, the linemen will be aware of that and they will run to the closest hash mark. They will automatically become your protection if you allow them to. But if you are running all over the place, it is very, very difficult for you to have coordinated blocking.

If you are creating interference in this situation, don't worry too much about your blocking technique. Be careful to the point that you don't clip your opponent or hit him with another kind of illegal block that could injure both you and your opponent, as well as set back your team. At the same time, remember that he is an offensive player who is suddenly on the defensive. He is just as unfamiliar with his new role as you are and just as startled to find himself there.

You can help your team a great deal just by getting in the way of any potential tackler. On an interception or fumble, you just want to occupy a guy so he won't make the tackle. Everybody is always excited in those situations and if you can get in your opponent's way, that's good. If you have a chance to take a shot and knock the daylights out of somebody, you do it. As long as it's a clean, legal shot. They take a shot at you when they're on offense; if you get a chance, you want to reciprocate.

After your football exercises are complete, stretch for at least 15 minutes.

Do your weight work, including 30 sit-ups and 30 push-ups.

THURSDAY

BREAKFAST: Kick off your morning with juice. Then have half a cantaloupe or honeydew melon. Complete your morning meal with a plate of waffles with syrup. Finish off with a fruit Danish, if you'd like.

▼

LUNCH: Today, choose one of your favorite pasta dishes, including ravioli, and enjoy it with tomato or red clam sauce. Include a side dish of broccoli, as well as a mixed green salad. Drink water or juice with your lunch.

▼

DINNER: We'll stick with Italian food tonight. Make your main course veal parmigiana with a side dish of white or brown rice. Add some carrots to your meal, plus dinner rolls or bread. Stay away from soda and other sweets. For dessert, try a plum or peach.

Warm up.
Stretch for 30 to 40 minutes.
Jog 2 miles. This is a light day. We just want to get some exercise in and break a sweat. Compared to what we've been doing, it's almost a day of rest. But to do nothing would set us back. We're going to get in some good-quality work, but it will be neither that long nor that difficult. Just as we want to be careful not to do too little, we want to make sure we don't do too much. That can be counterproductive at this stage of the program.
Stretch.
Finish the day with 30 sit-ups and 30 push-ups.

FRIDAY

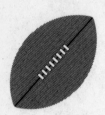

BREAKFAST: Start the week's final big workout day with a glass of juice and a grapefruit half or melon. Have a bowl of cold cereal—you should know by now what kind to eat—and French toast with syrup.

▼

LUNCH: Start off with a bowl of navy bean soup. With that, have a seafood salad sandwich or two on whole wheat bread. Include a mixed green salad and drink water or juice with your meal.

DINNER: Since it's Friday, I'll give you a choice. You can treat yourself to a lean sirloin steak or have grilled or baked salmon with lemon wedges.

Have wax or lima beans, plus potatoes or rice and dinner rolls. Have a banana or two for dessert.

Weigh yourself before working out.

Warm up.

Stretch for 30 to 40 minutes.

Jump rope for 10 to 15 minutes.

Run two half-miles at three-quarter speed, primarily to warm up the body for the sprint work that will follow.

Stretch hard.

Do two 300-yard shuttle runs.

Follow those with two 200-yard shuttle runs.

Finish up with five 100-yard sprints. These do not have to be at full speed; go about three-quarter speed. We're stressing the quality of our running here. Concentrate on keeping your form while you're running. Put in that extra effort. Training camp is just a month away and today you're getting a good indication of your condition. Don't cheat yourself.

Drink fluid-replacement beverages every 15 minutes or so.

Warm down and stretch.

Do your weight work, including 30 sit-ups and 30 push-ups.

After four weeks in the weight room, you should be noticeably stronger than you were when you began lifting weights. Your arm and leg muscles may be larger than they were. But keep in mind, you are working so hard in the weight room to help you become a better football player. You aren't in there to improve your looks or to turn yourself into a bodybuilder. You don't have to look like a champion weight lifter to be successful in football.

If you don't believe me, study Joe Montana the next time you watch the 49ers on television. If you look at him in street clothes or in shorts, you would never think he possesses the skills that he does.

Joe's not a very big guy—you would never think he's a great quarterback, because he's so small.

When you look at quarterbacks, you think of a guy like Terry Bradshaw, who was 6 feet 4 inches and about 200 pounds. Joe Montana is not Terry Bradshaw. But once he puts those pads on, he's a totally different man. He has very strong arms, he's very mobile and very smart. He knows how to win games and he knows how to make big plays.

I remember the first time I played him. It was in my rookie

season, 1984, in the play-offs in San Francisco. I was right out of college and I'd seen the guy on TV, but there he was, in person. During pre-game warm-ups I was looking at Montana and thinking to myself that he was not very big. In college, if a guy looks like Montana does, the first thing that goes through your mind is that you're going to cream him. Well, that isn't the case in the pros.

We certainly didn't clobber Montana that day. On one play, he was scrambling around trying to find an open receiver, when he took off running. He got past the linemen and linebackers. One of our safeties ran up to him and it looked like he was about to step out of bounds when he put a fake on the guy that fooled everybody and ran for 10 yards more.

When you play Montana, you have to be aware of all the tricks he can pull. He's the thinking man's quarterback and he knows how to win games.

No lead is safe with him in there. We discovered that painfully in the second game of the 1988 season. The Giants took a 17–13 lead when Lionel Manuel caught a touchdown pass with 1:21 remaining in the game.

That was much too much time to leave for Montana. He hit Jerry Rice on a 78-yard touchdown bomb that gave the 49ers a 20–17 victory. It proved once again that if you give Joe Montana a chance, he'll beat you.

It's a good lesson for young players to learn. The biggest and strongest players don't always come out on top. You have to play intelligently and you have to have an unyielding will to win.

THE WEEKEND

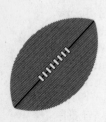

Eat well, drink healthful fluids, warm up, stretch, and soak.

W E E K 7

Relax. This week will not be as hard as last week was. You have worked hard and you deserve a little rest. If you have been following the program diligently, you should be in pretty good shape. But you don't want to peak too quickly. It's important that you have something left for pre-season practice.

We've been working very hard up to this point and we want to give our muscles a chance to relax. We don't want to burn out before camp; we need to give the muscles a break so that when we resume full-scale workouts next week, our muscles will still be responding in the way that they have up until this point. By the same token, we don't want to lose any of our conditioning with this light week. So, we're going to be doing some things, but not as much, to maintain our edge.

In addition to easing up on your running requirements this week, you should also lighten up a little on your weight work. Keep the same weight and do the same exercises, but do fewer repetitions. This will allow you to get your work in, while at the same time giving yourself a bit of a break. This will help give you the strength to go all out in the next two weeks leading up to training camp.

I would stress again, however, that it is important that you continue to stretch every day. We're going to start our final push toward pre-season practice next week, and one of the last things you want to get is a pulled muscle that will put you out of action.

Another important facet of the program that you should not change at all is your diet. Make sure you keep eating good foods and drinking healthful beverages. A decreased work load at the track and in the weight room is no reason to start eating junk food. You should maintain a healthful diet at all times. If you deviate now, you will surely pay for it next week, when we again increase the intensity of our workouts.

MONDAY

BREAKFAST: Begin the workout week with a glass of juice and a fruit cocktail. Follow that with waffles and syrup or honey. If you feel you need a bit more, have a sweet roll or English muffin.

▼

LUNCH: Start the noontime meal with a bowl of vegetable soup and crackers. This may be a relatively light work week, but I don't want to skimp on the carbohydrates. Let's eat stuffed shells with tomato sauce and a mixed green salad. Drink water or juice and complete your lunch with a bowl of Jell-O.

▼

DINNER: Tonight we'll have baked or broiled chicken with fresh carrots and red potatoes. Don't forget the dinner rolls. For dessert, eat apples, oranges, and/or grapes.

Weigh yourself before working out.
Warm up.
Stretch for 30 to 40 minutes.
Jump rope for 10 to 15 minutes.
Run a mile and a half with a football. It doesn't have to be full speed, but don't run less than three-quarter speed.
Warm down and stretch.
Do your weight work, remembering to do fewer repetitions. Make sure you do 30 sit-ups and 30 push-ups.

TUESDAY

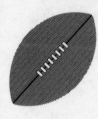

BREAKFAST: Start off with a glass of juice and a grapefruit half. Then have a bowl or two of healthful cold cereal, making sure to stay away from added sugar. Complement that with an English muffin or toast with honey.

▼

LUNCH: Have a bowl of chicken soup with rice or noodles. With that, we'll have a turkey club on whole wheat bread with potato salad and, of course, a tossed salad. Drink water, juice, or low-fat milk and have a piece of fruit for dessert.

▼

DINNER: Tonight we'll have spaghetti and meatballs or meat sauce, with mixed vegetables and rolls and bread. Drink water or juice with your meal. For dessert, eat a pear, peach, or banana.

Warm up.
Stretch for 30 to 40 minutes.
Work for at least 20 minutes on football drills.
If you feel like jogging for a mile or jumping rope for 10 or 15 minutes, then do it. But remember, the focus this week is on giving ourselves a rest while not losing any of our conditioning edge. Don't think that you're not doing enough and try to do too much. You'll be working hard enough over the final three weeks to make up for whatever break you're getting this week.

WEDNESDAY

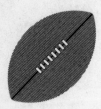

BREAKFAST: We'll begin today with a glass of juice and a cantaloupe or honeydew melon half. Then have a bowl or two of hot cereal, along with an English muffin and honey. Finish off the meal with a fruit Danish.

▼

LUNCH: Start off with a bowl of navy bean soup with crackers. Treat yourself to a couple of hamburgers today, though I would prefer that you not eat french fries with them. And make sure the ground beef is lean. Don't leave out the green salad. Drink water or juice with your meal and have some sherbet if you want dessert.

▼

DINNER: Tonight we'll eat manicotti with peas and carrots, plus rolls or bread. Add a salad if you'd like. Drink water or juice. For dessert, eat a banana or grapes.

Warm up, including 10 to 15 minutes of jumping rope.
Stretch for 30 to 40 minutes.
Run a half-mile at three-quarter speed.
Stretch to prepare your body for shorter-distance work.
Run ten 110-yard sprints with a three-quarter-speed stride.
Do 15 minutes of football drills. This week, begin working on your tackling technique (see below).
After you have finished your football exercises, jog a lap.
Stretch.
Do your weight work, remembering to cut back on the number of repetitions you do.
Finish with 30 sit-ups and 30 push-ups.
Proper tackling techniques is important for all football players. Defensive players, of course, use their tackling skills far more frequently than do offensive players. But all football players should know how to tackle properly. If you play on offense, you never know when you may have to bring down an opposing player who has intercepted a pass or recovered a fumble. In addition, your coach may place you on the punt or kickoff teams, where tackling skills

are crucial. Offensive players can reduce their risk of injury tremendously by learning how to tackle properly.

Never underestimate the importance of special teams. Good special teams help win a lot of games, while poor special teams can lose even more. If you are a good tackler, you can be an excellent special teams player. Speed is important, but it is not the key to your success.

A terrific special teams player on the Giants is Reyna Thompson, who we signed as a free agent before the 1989 season. Thompson was a cornerback who didn't see much action at that position. But he played on almost all of our special teams and always seemed to be among the first players down the field on punts and kickoffs. Because of his tackling skills, Thompson became one of the most important players on the team.

Among all the fine plays Reyna has made for us, one stands out to me. We were playing the Broncos on a snowy afternoon in Denver late in the 1989 season. With 1:24 remaining, we had a 14–7 lead when Sean Landeta punted the ball away for what would be the Broncos' last opportunity to win the game. Denver's best chance for victory was to get a long punt return that would give it good field position.

Ricky Nattiel caught the ball on the Broncos' 23-yard line. As soon as he tucked it away, Thompson, who had been hustling down the field, collided with Nattiel and sent him to the ground. It was a great football play that kept the Broncos pinned deep in their own territory. Denver never got closer than our 34 and we won a critical game by that 14–7 score. Reyna Thompson's hustle, as well as his ability to tackle, probably saved the game for us.

Of all the things I do on the football field, the most basic, and perhaps the most important, is tackling the offensive man with the ball. From my perspective, tackling is the bare essence of football. That's what the game boils down to—tackling and blocking. As a defensive player, the bottom line for me is making the tackle. No matter what you do or what you're good at, you have to be a good tackler.

If you are not a good tackler, your role will be minimized. You will likely become a situation player and you won't see much action with the game on the line. Your importance to the team will decrease, because linebackers are supposed to be the best tacklers on the team. If you want to be a linebacker, and you can't tackle, you'd better start looking for a different position. Quickly.

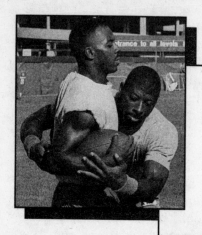

On every tackle keep your head up, your eyes open, and your arms around the ballcarrier to drive him to the ground.

What makes a good tackle is not the hit that knocks somebody out, but the hit that brings somebody down. To be that type of tackler, you need to follow my three basic rules for a good, effective tackle: (1) Keep your head up; (2) keep your eyes open; (3) wrap your arms around the ballcarrier and drive him to the ground.

By following these rules in 1989 I had only ten missed tackles, less than one a game.

The first two rules go hand-in-hand. It does you no good to keep your eyes open if you're looking down at the ground. You can't see the running back anyway.

More important, *it is extremely unsafe to attempt to make a tackle with your head down.* Many serious injuries occur in football for the simple reason that a player doesn't keep his head up. If your head is down, your neck is in a weak position. With your eyes looking down, the only things you can see are your shoes and the ground around them. You can't see the play developing and you won't have any idea who or what is headed your way. You certainly won't be able to see the ballcarrier, who is the man you want to tackle. If your head is down he could walk by you, because you won't have a clue where to look for him.

Keeping your head up won't help if your eyes don't stay open. I have teammates who miss tackles because they close their eyes as the ballcarrier approaches. When I watch football on television, I see college and other professional players miss tackles they should make because they didn't keep their eyes open. Keeping your head up and your eyes open allows you to do a lot of other things, like seeing your opponent and where he's going. If he tries to fake you out, you will be able to adjust.

It's human nature to close your eyes on contact. Imagine if you're at bat in a baseball game and the pitcher throws the ball right at you. You are not going to stand there and watch that ball hit your body. You're going to close your eyes, duck your head, and try to hop out of the way.

The same mentality applies in football. But there are significant differences. In football, as in baseball, you are the aggressor. But in football you have protection, such as shoulder pads and a helmet with a face guard. The chances that another player's helmet is going to go through your helmet are almost nonexistent, so you can keep your eyes open without fear of injury.

If you close your eyes, you are going to drop your head. As we've already discussed, nothing good happens when your head drops. Your reaction will be the same as it would be if that errant baseball was coming at you. In baseball, you would legitimately be trying to avoid contact. But in football, you should be initiating it. That's hard to do if you can't see what you're trying to hit.

Keeping your eyes open during a tackle is something you can practice, to a degree. You can work on your tackling technique with a tackling dummy and get in the habit of leaving your eyes open that way. It's a matter of doing it over and over and telling yourself that you have to do it this way. Because a dummy doesn't move, you can easily convince yourself to knock the crap out of it while keeping your eyes wide open.

It's a little different with a moving target, especially when that target is a large back running toward you at full speed. With a moving target in a game situation, you have to tell yourself to keep your eyes open and your head up, and once you do that, over and over again, then it becomes second nature.

Step three in tackling is wrapping up the ballcarrier. Put your arms around him and grab hold of something. It's difficult sometimes to make a chest-to-chest tackle, with your helmet underneath his. That is considered a perfect tackle. You can't always make that kind of tackle, because running backs don't make a habit of squaring up so you can easily bring them down.

Since the offensive player usually refuses to cooperate, you have to use your shoulder pads to hit him, then wrap your arms around him and grab hold of him. If you can wrap your arms around a

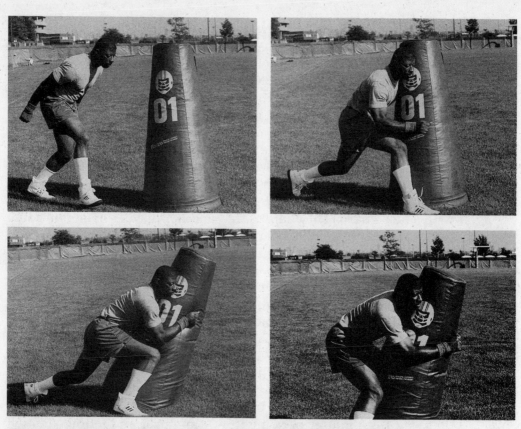

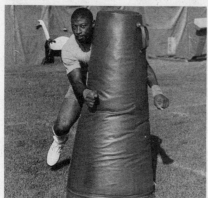 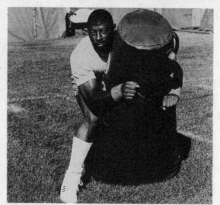

Tackling is one of football's most basic skills and you must follow three rules if you are going to succeed. The first is to keep your head up, the second is to keep your eyes open, and the third is to wrap your arms around the ballcarrier and keep them there until he is on the ground. If you neglect even one of these rules, you will miss a lot of tackles.

ballcarrier, lock one of your hands around the opposite wrist, so he won't be able to escape your grip. Once you've taken care of that step, drive your legs and push him backward.

When you get the basics down, it's important to know, that in order to be a good tackler, you have to be the one to deliver the blow. You can't be a catcher. You have to be a hitter. If you see a guy running very hard, you have to run very hard so you can be the primary force at the point of contact. If not, then you will be tumbling backward, not him.

Good position and preparation are also important. Positioning has to be done on the run. You have to have a sense of depth perception and you must know what angle the ballcarrier is taking, as well as where your defensive help is. It does you no good to break down for a tackle too early. By breaking down, I mean getting into a hitting position. If you do that when the offensive player is 5 yards away, and he sees you sitting there, he's going to run in the opposite direction.

You have to get yourself to within 2 or 3 feet of the man with the ball before you get into a hitting position. That minimizes the running back's options. If you're 2 to 3 feet away from the guy, you can still change direction if he cuts. You're not too far away to make contact if he tries to put a move on you.

If the running back has a lot of room to work, then you know that his options are greater than yours. You have to cut down his options and give him one way to go and force him that way. If you know that all of your help is on the inside of you, then at any cost you want to force this guy to the inside. If this ballcarrier is faster than you, you're not in trouble, because he is running straight back into the teeth of the defense.

There's nothing cowardly about jumping on a ballcarrier's back if he is lower than you. That will enable you to keep your head up. Because if he's lower than you, and you have to duck your head to get under his, chances are you're going to suffer an injury. You can't hit what you can't see. You can't hit a fastball with your eyes closed and you can't tackle a ballcarrier if you can't see him.

Certain running backs are harder for me to tackle than others. One is Herschel Walker. When I see him running at me, I don't know where I want to attack him. I would like to get him on the smallest part of his body, which is around his legs. But not on his thighs, because they're extremely big and powerful. And I don't want to take him up high: I won't be able to wrap him up, because his

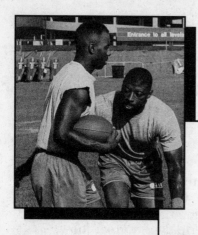

Don't try to strip the ball at the expense of a good tackle.

shoulder pads are so big. He has good upper body movement when he runs with the ball. And I don't want to run into him head on, because he's just as big and strong as I am.

A head-on collision with Herschel makes it a 50–50 proposition as to who is going to go backward. I would rather not take that chance. If Walker has the ball and is bearing down on me, I'd better follow my top two rules or he could very easily inflict a lot of damage on me. A lot of times with Herschel, I just try to grab a piece of him and wait for help, because he's so strong—he's like a huge truck motoring through there. I just want to make sure I get hold of something before the cavalry arrives.

As I mentioned before, Roger Craig is also tough to bring down. Roger is not a real big guy, only about 195 to 200 pounds. It's always best to try to tackle him before he gets a full head of steam. If he gains momentum, it's really hard to tackle him down low, because his legs are very powerful and he brings his knees up extremely high.

I think the best running back in the league today is Barry Sanders of the Detroit Lions. He has great speed and a low center of gravity, as well as very, very powerful legs, which makes it difficult to tackle him below the waist. When you go up against a guy like Sanders, you almost have to abandon everything you've learned about tackling the ballcarrier around the waist. You have to tackle Sanders high, because you're not going to trip him up by taking a shot at him down low.

We played the Lions at Giants Stadium early in the 1989 season, Sanders' rookie year. Detroit was knocking on our door, with a third-and-one from our 4-yard line. Barry got the ball and broke through the line of scrimmage. I didn't have the correct angle to make a perfect form tackle, but I had a chance to knock him over. I hit him what I thought was a hard shot in his legs. He stopped, restarted, and went on into the end zone for a touchdown.

It was a great play on his part, as well as a perfect example of his tremendous leg strength and balance. Another asset of Barry's is that he has excellent hands. The Lions use the run-and-shoot passing attack, so there are games during the course of every season when Sanders won't get a lot of handoffs. But they throw the ball to him on screen passes and flare passes. He does a great job catching the ball, and once he gets it, he runs well with it. Barry isn't the fastest running back in the league, but he has breakaway speed. He can get through the line of scrimmage in a hurry. He gets a very good start from his stance in the backfield to the line of scrimmage. When the ball is snapped, he gets to where he is supposed to be in a hurry.

Another running back who I think shows a great deal of promise and will cause headaches for tacklers like myself for many years is Tim Worley of the Pittsburgh Steelers. He's a combination of Eric Dickerson and Herschel Walker. Worley is tall and he has great moves for a runner his size, good acceleration to the hole. He's tough to bring down in the open field, because he's so big. He also has good speed, unusual in a player that large.

Curt Warner of the Los Angeles Rams presents different problems. You don't know which way he's going to run. When he was with Seattle, the Seahawks had plays designed for him to run in a specific hole, but there was no guarantee he was going to be there once he got the ball in his hands. He would start running into that hole and end up somewhere else.

Warner is difficult to bring down in the open field, because he doesn't take a lot of punishment. He doesn't give you a lot of body to hit and he can squirm for an extra yard.

But as difficult as Walker, Craig, and Warner are as running backs, the same rules apply in trying to tackle all three: Keep your head up. Keep your eyes open. Wrap your arms and drive the ballcarrier into the ground.

Where you make a tackle is also very important. It doesn't do your team much good if you bring a ballcarrier down in the end

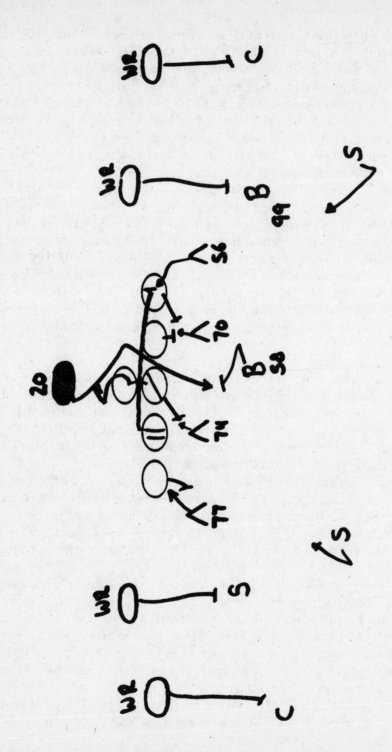

Barry Sanders of the Detroit Lions somehow made his way through traffic and stayed on his feet after I gave him a hard shot in the legs, to score a touchdown on this play early in the 1989 season.

zone. If you make a tackle at the line of scrimmage, it's great. If you make it behind the line of scrimmage, it's even better.

Several times during a game, you will be tempted to go for the ball instead of the ballcarrier. The runner will appear to be holding the ball loosely, holding it as if getting hit is the last thing on his mind. Because it looks as if he's being careless with the ball, you may think that by lunging at it you will be able to force a fumble.

Unless you are absolutely, positively, 100 percent certain you can jar the ball loose, I strongly recommend that you concentrate your efforts on the runner and not the ball. Chances are very good that the running back or end will be in better control of the ball than you think he is. If he is, and you lunge for the football, you will have nothing more than an embarrassing missed tackle.

You may think you have a clear shot at knocking the football loose, but that can be very deceptive. When two bodies are traveling at a high rate of speed, a lot of things can change in a short period of time. One of them is your seemingly easy forced fumble. I've found that most most of the times I go for the ball at the expense of the ballcarrier, I get neither. The result, of course, is that the ballcarrier gains a lot of yardage.

Sometimes it is imperative for me to try and jar the ball loose. Most of those times are near the end of a game in which the Giants are trailing. The clock is running out and we have to get the ball back. We have no choice but to go for the ball.

In rare instances, I focus on the ball at times other than in those desperate situations. Oddly enough, I was once successful in separating the ball from Barry Sanders.

The Lions had a first-and-10 on our 12-yard line when Sanders ran a draw play. I was trailing the play from the side, reached my hand in there and grabbed the tip of the ball. It flipped up in the air and landed right in my lap.

I made sure to tackle Sanders first. I took my outside arm and wrapped it around his waist. Then I took my other arm, jarred the ball, and took it out.

The rule I follow is that if I have a chance to make the tackle, I do that first and try to strip the ball simultaneously. I never go for the strip first unless I absolutely have no other choice, which can happen when the ballcarrier is out of my reach and I can't do anything but try to dive for the ball. It's best to wrap one arm around the ballcarrier and then try to pull the ball out. If you don't succeed in getting the ball, you still have him tied up and you can bring him down.

I don't advise just going for the ball, especially if you're in a position to make a tackle. If you go for the ball and you miss, it means extra yardage for the offensive team. That is not what you're out there for.

The Open Field Tackle

Probably the most difficult tackle to make in football is the open field tackle. The open field is where the good tacklers are identified and the bad ones are exposed. In the open field, there's only you, the ballcarrier, and air. If you can bring the ballcarrier down in that situation, then you are a good tackler.

One of the best teachers I've had in this endeavor is Bill Belichick, my defensive coordinator on the Giants. He taught me that there are several steps required to execute a successful open field tackle. The first thing you must do is close the distance between yourself and the ballcarrier. The more room in which the offensive player has to maneuver, the more difficult it's going to be for you to catch him and bring him to the ground.

It sounds strange, but you have to wait while not really waiting. If you have a 20-yard distance between the runner and you, the first thing you want to do is close down that runner's options. When he's 20 yards away, the runner knows he can do just about anything he wants: he has the room and the advantage. You have to take both away by running as hard as you can for 10 yards. But that's still too early to break down. Get yourself under control until you're 5 yards away, then break down and prepare to make the tackle at 2 or 3 yards. By being under control, I mean that you should still be closing the distance between yourself and the running back. Once you're close enough to make contact, you make a good form tackle on the run.

When you are caught in the middle of the field like this, and you're cutting off the distance between the ballcarrier and you, I strongly suggest that you focus on his hips or waist. The most stable part of a runner is his hips. Once his hips move, then that's the direction the runner's going to take. His feet and head can move much more easily, and if you stay focused on either of them, you are more susceptible to a fake. So it's best to keep a bead on the runner's

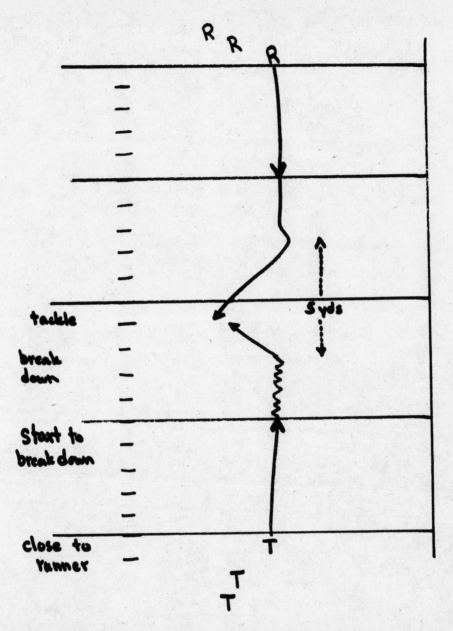

You can't commit yourself too early when you're trying to make an open field tackle. If you do, the ballcarrier will see it and easily avoid you. You have to wait until you're five yards from the ballcarrier before you begin to get into tackling position. Maintain self-control and don't attempt the tackle until you are two or three yards away.

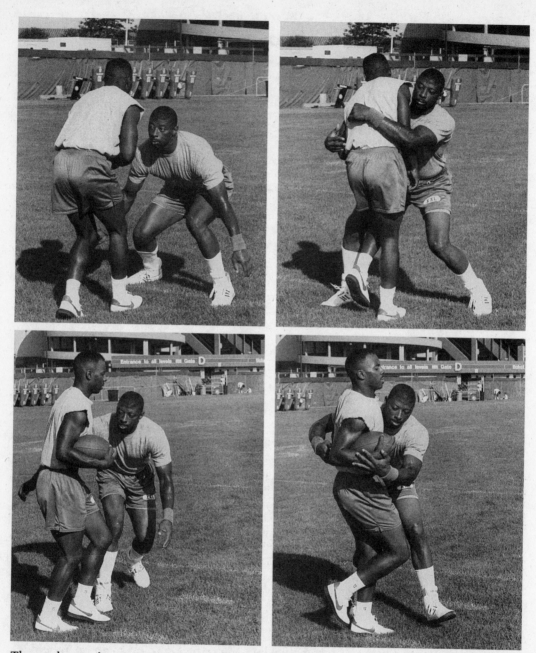

These photos demonstrate how close you should be before you try to take down the ballcarrier in an open-field tackling situation. If you try to tackle him earlier, you'll be retracing your steps, because he will have slipped past you and back into the open field.

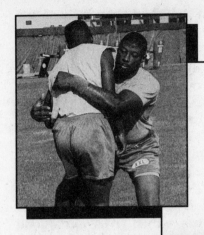

In an open-field situation, cut down the space between you and the ballcarrier before getting into tackling position.

waist or hips, because they will determine which way that runner is going to go.

On occasion, a defensive player closes the distance so fast that the running back becomes confused. The back can't decide what to do and runs directly into the defender. It makes the defender's job easier, but a defensive player can't count on a running back to lose his poise so that he can make the play.

Sometimes during a game, you will receive help making a tackle and your teammates won't even be involved. That aid will come from the sideline. If you are chasing a ballcarrier who is between the sideline and you, run at an angle that will force the ballcarrier to indicate which way he's going to have to go. He will have to head toward the sideline or back in the direction you are coming from. If the sideline is to your left, you take an inside-out position running. That would put your right shoulder to his inside, or left, shoulder, and your shoulder should be splitting his body, pushing his right side to the sideline.

As you close the distance, turn and make sure you end up in a squared-up position, or face-to-face with the ballcarrier. But that's only after you've closed the field down on him and forced him to go in one direction. If you end up in a face-to-face position too far away, then he can go either way.

In a game, I have to be able to make one-on-one tackles on backs or tight ends who are bigger than I am. Strength and football ability help, but they alone can't win the battle for me. When

Herschel Walker, Eric Dickerson, or James Wilder are speeding toward me, there's no place to hide. Those kinds of backs can be just as strong and just as athletic as I am. Smaller backs, such as Tony Dorsett and Stump Mitchell, present different kinds of problems. They are so quick they can give you a move or two and be by you before you have a chance to get your arms into tackling position. Strength doesn't help very much if you can't catch anything to hold on to.

A cardinal rule with a big back like Walker or a tight end is to try and not tackle them high. With their great upper body strength, it's like grabbing a train and holding on while they take you for a ride. Herschel is a perfect example. He has incredible upper body strength. But he doesn't have great moves, which gives you a good opportunity to try and take his legs out from under him.

The key to stopping a guy like Herschel Walker is to get to him early, before he has a full head of steam. After about five steps he really has it going, and then you have to aim for his legs. And you have to make sure you wrap him up, because he keeps those legs going pretty good.

When a running back, large or small, is coming at you in the open field, that is the time to rehearse in your head exactly what you're going to do. Any indecision at the point of attack can result in a lot of things, all of them embarrassing. Such as being completely trampled, getting up, and watching the referee spot the ball 10 yards past your body. Or getting your helmet knocked off, because the runner shot a forearm in your chest and brought it up through your helmet. Or being run over and knowing the only reason the guy was brought down was because he stumbled while stepping into your chest. When you see a guy like this coming right at you, focus on his waist or hips. If he's close enough, you can keep your eyes focused on his legs just below his kneecaps. If you hit him there, you know he'll go down.

When I am tackling someone, I try to use as much of my shoulder pads as possible. The backs and ends I try to stop are so powerful that an arm tackle wouldn't bring them down. My head has to be in the right position. If it isn't, I could get hurt.

Finally, it's important for a player in an open-field tackling position to convince himself that he's not going to be scared. Knowing all this comes from repetition, preparation, and confidence. All the embarrassing scenes I described have happened to me. If young players follow my rules, they could avoid having these things happen to them. They will be able to bring down the Herschel Walkers of their league.

The proudest moment for me in making an open field tackle was when I brought down Gary Clark, a fleet little receiver for the Washington Redskins, in a game during the 1987 season at Giants Stadium. It was right before halftime. Clark caught a swing pass on my side, which left me alone with this fast, shifty receiver. If I wasn't careful, he could be past me before I had a chance to blink my eyes.

He was running toward me, and I knew he had great moves, including a spin move that could corkscrew a defender into the ground. Clark was close to the sideline and I was on the inside, about 15 yards away from him when our duel began. One mistake on my part and the Redskins would have 6 points. I was running as fast as I could to cut the distance down to at least 5 yards. Fortunately, he didn't see me coming.

I got the distance closed down to about 5 yards, where I got my body under control. At that point, he surely knew I was there and had to declare which way he was going to go. He tried a few juke steps which didn't fool me at all, because I was looking at his hips all the way, not at his head and shoulders. Clark made another move. I was right there. My head was up. I wrapped him up right around his knees. I think my helmet was right around his waist. I made what I thought was a great hit, and after we were getting up off the ground, he said, "That was a good tackle." That made me feel good, coming from Gary Clark, because he's so elusive and so hard to bring down.

Whether you're facing a powerful back like Walker or an elusive player like Clark, the worst thing you can do in attempting to make an open field tackle is to lunge at the runner. It's like flying off a diving board. You have no solid base and no chance to change direction if there's a sudden move by the runner.

Body control is the key. You make the runner commit, but once he does, you have to be in the position to make the tackle. It does no good to make the guy commit in one direction or another if he just keeps going. And that often happens if you don't have your body under control.

Of course, I have had my share of missed tackles, embarrassing moments, and plays I would just as soon forget. The one that stands out most vividly was when I didn't bring down Randall Cunningham, the Philadelphia Eagles' quarterback, in a Monday Night

Football game in 1988. It's a play that has made a lot of highlight tapes, but it was a lowlight for me.

The Giants were leading 3–0 early in the second period. Philadelphia had taken possession on its own 20 and driven all the way down to our 4-yard line, where it was third-and-goal. If we could hold them, the Eagles would get no better than a field goal, which would tie the game.

Cunningham took the snap and rolled to his right, only to find me standing directly in front of him. My body was under control. He set to pass and had nowhere to go. I went right at him in an attempt to make the tackle and hit him squarely in the knees. Because I was so close to him, I didn't think I needed to keep driving my legs. I just lunged right into him.

His legs went completely out from under him. The only thing that kept him from going down was that I didn't keep my legs driving. But once I felt his legs leave the ground, I thought he was down and at that point, I let him go. Cunningham, however, got one arm down on the ground and used the ball as a cushion, which prevented either of his knees from touching the turf. Had one of his knees touched, that would have ended the play. He pushed himself up with his free arm and threw the ball to Jimmie Giles for a shocking touchdown. I dropped to the ground in frustration.

That was a great play on Cunningham's part. I tried to wrap him up, but he used his tremendous athletic ability to prevent me from doing just that. If I ever have to repeat that play, I may have to do it the same way. Next time, though, I would try to totally crush him.

It was somewhat embarrassing, but I think there're a lot of players who would have suffered a similar fate on that play, because Cunningham has so much talent.

For several weeks after that game, I'd go out and people would ask me, "How did Randall Cunningham make that play?" They'd look at me and say, "You had him down." The only thing I can say is that sometimes those things happen in football. You just don't want them to happen and turn into a touchdown.

I watched the tape of that play over and over again with my coaches. They thought that the tackle I tried to make would have brought most players down. I have made almost identical tackles and put players on the ground. But that time I didn't and the only way I will be able to rectify the situation is to get him again. I doubt it would be the exact situation, but I look forward to making a spectacular play against him.

You practice tackling skills and prepare yourself for your own spectacular plays. Get a tackling dummy from your local sporting goods store or borrow one from your school. Set it up in the middle of the field and run at it from different angles. Even though the dummy doesn't move, you can work on the basics of tackling, such as having your head up, your eyes open, and your legs driving. Work on wrapping and squeezing your arms around your opponent.

You can use the bag to simulate different game situations. Put the bag at a 45-degree angle and run toward it. Get in good position with your head up and eyes open and drive through the bag. Go behind the bag and simulate a tackle from behind. You can also have a friend hold the bag. As you break down and get in a good tackling position, have him move the bag from side to side. Once he lets go, you have to be in proper position to hit the bag.

Tackling is a vital skill for any football player. Work hard at it, because good tacklers are valuable to any football team.

THURSDAY

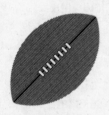

BREAKFAST: A glass of juice and the fruit of your choice. Try blueberries, strawberries, or raspberries if you're looking for a change of pace. We'll move on to two or three scrambled eggs with potatoes or grits, and a muffin, bagel, or toast with honey.

▼

LUNCH: Today we'll have a bowl of vegetable or lentil soup with crackers. We'll continue with a hot turkey sandwich on the bread of your choice, mashed potatoes, and a green salad. Drink fluid-replacement beverages and have a piece of fruit for dessert.

▼

DINNER: Let's eat a lean veal chop, white or brown rice, and asparagus. If you don't like asparagus, pick another vegetable. Make sure you eat dinner rolls or bread, and stay away from soda. For dessert, have a bowl of ice milk with some of the leftover berries from breakfast.

Warm up, including jumping rope for 10 to 15 minutes.

Stretch for 30 to 40 minutes.

Run four 220-yard sprints at a strider's pace. I'm not asking you to do a lot today, so don't cheat yourself on what you are supposed to do.

If you take shortcuts here, you're going to pay for them next week.

Do at least 20 minutes of football drills, touching all areas, but concentrating most on those that pertain to your position.

Finish with 30 sit-ups and 30 push-ups.

FRIDAY

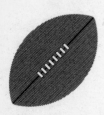

BREAKFAST: Kick off with a glass of your favorite juice and a fruit cocktail. Then eat pancakes, either plain or blueberry, with syrup. Eat ham slices with those, if you'd like.

▼

LUNCH: Let's keep it simple for this final workout day. Have a bowl of clam chowder or tomato soup. With that, have a tuna fish sandwich or two on rolls or bread. Make sure you have a green salad. Complete your lunch with a bowl of Jell-O, with or without fruit.

▼

DINNER: Enjoy your final treat of the light week with prime ribs of beef. Of course, you must make certain it's lean by cutting away any excess fat. Have a baked potato with that, as well as stir-fry vegetables fried in olive oil. Don't forget the dinner rolls. For dessert, eat ice milk or sherbet.

Remember, we are going to pick up the pace again next week.

Warm up.

Stretch for 30 to 40 minutes.

Run a half-mile at three-quarter speed.

Do two 330-yard runs and two 220-yard runs, all at three-quarter speed. If you play a position that requires you to handle the football, hold a ball while running.

Drink fluid-replacement beverages at regular intervals.

Stretch.

Do your weight work, remembering to cut back on the number of repetitions you do. Finish with 30 sit-ups and 30 push-ups.

THE WEEKEND

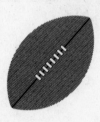

Eat well, drink plenty of fluids, warm up, stretch, and soak.

At this point in the program, I am thinking more and more about the coming season. I start to formulate a list of goals that I want to achieve. And I begin to plot how I'm going to play some of the opponents I am certain to face.

One player I will probably be up against for many years is Troy Aikman, the Dallas quarterback who was a rookie in 1989 after being the first pick in the draft.

Aikman is an extremely impressive quarterback. He has a very strong, accurate arm. One of the things coaches look for in a quarterback is whether he can throw a 25-yard in-cut. There's a lot of traffic in that part of the field. A quarterback has to have the right velocity on the ball, he has to throw it the correct height to get it over the intermediate defenders, and the pass has to come down at the right time so the receiver can get it when he's not hung up in the air, where a defender can give him a vicious shot. Aikman throws that pass as well as I've seen it thrown.

Early in my career, I spent a lot of time pondering how I was going to stop another Cowboy, Tony Dorsett.

Dorsett used to give us fits. He was a slashing runner, but he also had a lot of shake-and-bake in him. Dorsett had great acceleration. One of the qualities he had that I haven't seen in another runner was the ability to cut on one step. He could be running in one direction, plant his foot, and start running in the other direction with just one step. It usually takes a player at least a couple of steps to gather his body and start moving in the opposite direction. Dorsett could do it with a single step, because he had such a low center of gravity when he ran.

Next week, we begin the final push toward training camp. Prepare yourself this weekend. And think about the great things you want to accomplish on the football field.

W E E K

You had a little breather last week, to give you a chance to regain the strength in your legs. This week, we're going to step up our effort a notch as we begin the final push toward training camp. We're also going to start cutting down your distances in running. From now until the end of the program, you will be running distances that are more closely tailored to your work on the football field.

We have three weeks to go before the beginning of training camp. When you get there, I want you to have a body that is ready to take on the grueling demands of the football season.

To reach that goal, I want you to give your maximum effort over these final three weeks. We're going to work a little harder than we have up to this point. We're adding a few more drills and/or repetitions to drills we have already been doing.

To guard against injury when you are putting in that little extra effort, you must stretch properly. The last thing you want now is a pulled muscle. This is the final drive toward the season. Don't let yourself come up short.

MONDAY

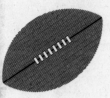

BREAKFAST: Begin the week with a glass of juice and a cantaloupe half. Then eat a bowl or two of honey-sweetened hot cereal, with an English muffin, bagel, or two pieces of toast.

▼

LUNCH: A bowl of vegetable soup with crackers, followed by barbecued, baked, or broiled chicken. Include a mixed green salad and a roll or two. Drink water or juice with your meal and have a bowl of Jell-O if you want dessert.

▼

DINNER: Tonight we'll have veal parmigiana, with a side dish of spaghetti and tomato sauce. Have some Brussels sprouts or broccoli with that, as well as dinner rolls or bread. Drink water or juice and have peaches or plums for dessert.

Warm up, including 5 minutes of jumping rope.

Stretch for 30 to 40 minutes, taking extra care that all muscles are properly stretched.

While carrying a football, run a half-mile at three-quarter speed.

Do five 220-yard runs at full speed. Try not to take more than 30 seconds between runs.

Take a brief rest and drink some fluids. Then run five 110-yard runs, also at full stride. When you do the 110s, sprint, walk back to the starting line, and sprint again. Don't waste time before or after the running.

Run a half-mile at three-quarter speed while again carrying a football. You will probably be a bit fatigued at this point, so concentrate hard and don't drop the ball.

Do 30 minutes of football drills. They should be directly related to what you will be doing in training camp. These can include agility exercises, catching passes, blocking drills, or pass drops.

After you finish your football drills, warm down and stretch.

Do your weight work.

Finish with 30 sit-ups and 30 push-ups.

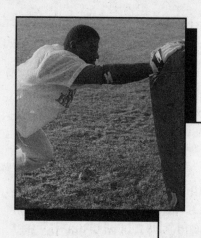

Use your hands to create separation between the blocker and you.

Fending Off Blockers

Last week, I taught you how to tackle properly. Now I'd like you to begin working on another facet of football that is extremely important: fending off blockers. The tackling skills you learned last week won't do you much good if you can't get away from the player whose job it is to keep you away from the ballcarrier.

The key to fending off an offensive player who is attempting to block you is to use your hands first. This creates the separation that enables you to get rid of the blocker and still have room to make the tackle, if the running back is close behind his interference.

A tandem that I had to contend with for many seasons was tackle Luis Sharpe and running back Stump Mitchell of the Phoenix Cardinals. Mitchell had great moves. But the number one thing a defensive player must be aware of is that the ballcarrier is going to go in the opposite direction from where he is. If you are on the outside of a blocker like Sharpe, then the running back, such as Mitchell, is going to cut back to the inside. The blocker is trying to form a wall and the runner is trying to use it as protection to advance as far as he can.

As a defensive player, you must get in a square position so that you can go either way on the blocker. By using your hands and creating a separation, you can throw that blocker off in either direction. Sometimes those guys are pretty hard to throw around. But you want to create a stalemate where you can move laterally, either left or right. If you fail to use your hands in the situation and you go in and try to use your forearm, then it's your body against his body. In both professional and collegiate football, the offensive linemen are very sneaky about grabbing hold of you and hooking your elbow inside of their arm. It's impossible to get away from them. To prevent that, you have to use your hands to separate yourself from them.

There will be other plays when your responsibility won't be to make the play, but to make sure that the play goes in a certain direction. In that case, always be alert. There's no rule that says you can't run to the other side of the field to help make a play.

For example, I am usually the left outside linebacker in the Giants' defense. On many plays, it is my job to keep the play inside of me, to my right. In that situation, I want to take on a blocker with my right shoulder and forearm. When doing so, I try to make sure that my left hand is free, just in case the running back is trying to force himself outside. By keeping my left arm free and showing that I am outside of the blocker, the running back will be forced to declare which way he's going to go. Chances are if he sees half of your body outside of his blocker, then he's going to go inside or you're going to force him to go inside. That, of course, was your responsibility in the first place.

Once you're in a position to force a play to go one way or the other, you still want to have enough room to shed the blocker. You do that with what we call a *drop step*. A drop step is simply taking the blocker on with one shoulder or the other. For example, if you're using your right shoulder, you have to use what is known as the *flipper*. That's taking your forearm and putting it right up into the blocker's chest. You use that forearm to create separation and neutralize the blocker's momentum. You get the separation by flipping the forearm up into your opponent's chest. Then you take your free hand and grab hold of the opposite pad. Pull with your free hand and turn the other shoulder with your forearm in the direction you're pulling. As you're doing that, you take the foot on the side of the aggressive forearm, in this case the right, and slide it outside the blocker.

An effective drop step is very similar to the technique a matador uses in a bullfight. As you're pulling, you're sliding the foot in the opposite direction. That clears your body from the blocker and puts you in a position to make the tackle.

When you're fending off a blocker, you have to deliver the blow;

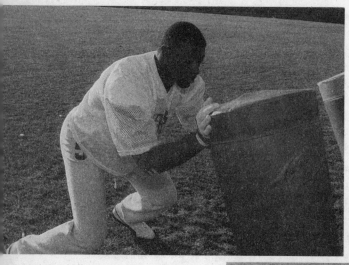

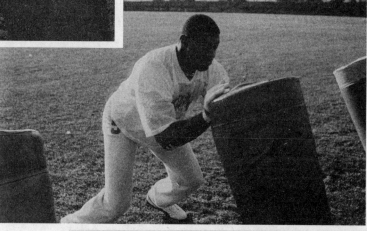

A defensive player has to be able to shed blockers by using his hands. You should practice taking on a blocker or pushing off on a tackling dummy or blocking shed. Always fight to keep your hands free.

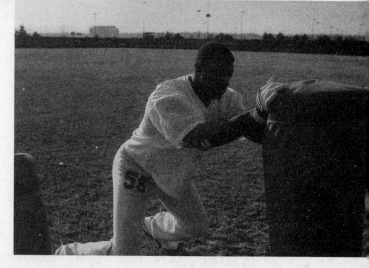

you can't absorb it. You have to deliver the blow with your shoulder and forearm. Once you've stalemated the blocker, you must take your free hand, the one that's outside the blocker, grab his shoulder pad and flip him down. It's almost like taking your forearm, pushing the blocker into your free hand so that you can go back inside for the block.

Remember, this all happens after the running back has declared which way he is going to go, or you have forced the play to go in the direction that you want.

Take again, for example, a situation where I'm lined up on the left and Mitchell is running a sweep to my side behind Sharpe. If the defense the coaches have designated calls for me to turn the play inside, I must try to get on Sharpe's outside shoulder. By no means do I want to be hooked by Luis Sharpe. That means I cannot allow Sharpe to get outside of my left leg. If I was playing the right side and he was coming at me in the same situation, I would have to prevent him from getting outside of my right leg.

To achieve my goal, I have to pursue the blocker at an angle from which Sharpe cannot reach my outside arm. You can't free-lance a path toward the blocker; you have to take a definite route relative to where the blocker is running. You can't keep widening your path. If that happens, you will wind up on the sideline and the running back will have a big alley to sail through. The key is to attack the blocker instead of letting him attack you.

If you're on the left side, you must attack him with your right

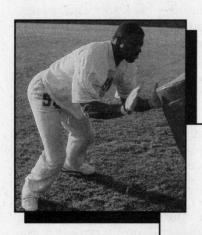

Deliver the blow when shedding a blocker; don't absorb it.

forearm and shoulder. Do this right away and, preferably, do it in the backfield behind the line of scrimmage. Don't wait for the blocker to come to you. Deliver a blow. But, it's not like jumping off a diving board. You can't just lunge into a guy.

A lot of the good running backs in the NFL today will start out with an inside running route and head right back outside. So you have to take a position where you can deliver a blow to the blocker, reach a stalemate, and then create separation.

That's where the drop step comes in. Remember, your primary objective is not to fight off the blocker. No one is going to notice your skirmish with the blocker if you don't tackle the runner, or if you don't create enough of a disturbance so that your teammates can stop him. Once you slip the blocker, you have to be able to fall back in and make the play, or at least help out on the play.

In the play I described, I know my primary objective is to tackle Mitchell, but the first thing I have to do is take care of Sharpe. The worst thing you can do is ignore the blocker and think that you're going to give him the slip easily to make the play on the running back. The running back is going to be watching his blocker and he's going to scamper away from you.

At the same time, you need to know where the running back is in relation to his blocker. If he's too close, there are times when you can deliver a blow to the blocker and the ballcarrier will run right into his blocker's back. That's one way to finish off a play.

Many times, the defense doesn't call for me to turn a sweep back toward the inside. My job is then to string the play out. By that I mean that my objective is to force the running back to wander from sideline to sideline instead of turning upfield toward the goal line.

If Sharpe is pulling around the corner and my responsibility is to direct Mitchell toward the sideline, he's going to try to hook me by getting outside of my outside arm. If he succeeds, Mitchell will be able to get past me, turn the corner, and head upfield. I have to get in a position that is almost head up, but slightly outside, because that's where the play is going. I take my hands and place them right inside of the blocker's shoulders, almost on his chest. You have to have a base under him, or you'll be in danger of getting pushed so far out that the play will succeed by running inside of you.

Once you place your hands securely on the lineman, immediately focus your eyes on the running back. The running back then is going to have to declare because he'll see the stalemate between the lineman and you. Ideally, the back would like to outrun you to the corner. But by having your hands on the lineman, you have created a standoff and you can throw the lineman in the direction opposite to that which the running back is going. By doing that, you are in a position to make the play or even force it out of bounds.

It is important to remember that when you have your hands on the lineman, you have to neutralize his movement. Simply putting your hands on him is not going to stop him, nor will it do anything to slow down the ballcarrier. You have to have some force behind it.

The drop step is also very important for inside linebackers. In the middle, the blockers are coming straight at you and you're frequently going to have to use your shoulder and forearm. In that case, it's crucial for an inside linebacker to know whether his responsibility is to turn the ball inside or outside. Once you've done that, you have to shed the blocker by using the drop-step technique.

All good inside linebackers are good drop-steppers or are very good at shedding blockers. Inside, you very seldom get a chance to use your hands when a play and/or a blocker is coming straight at you. There's only a distance of 3 or 4 yards between the blocker and you, and the running back is right behind the blocker.

Sometimes a linebacker will respond to an oncoming blocker by dropping down and hitting him in the legs, thus eliminating the blocker in this fashion. The Redskins have a play they often run in which the running back takes a jab step in one direction, then comes back to the opposite side. The purpose of the jab step is to give the guard and tackle on the opposite side an opportunity to get in front of the runner and block.

If we're playing the Redskins, guard Raleigh McKenzie and tackle Joe Jacoby will be pulling and bearing down on me. I know that neither of those guys has a great deal of agility when they start moving fast in one direction. So I take my outside shoulder and drive it right into the lead blocker's (McKenzie's) thigh. By continuing to move my feet, I cause him to stop, slow down, or fall down. The guy who's trailing behind him (Jacoby) will run right into him.

This accomplishes several things, all beneficial to the defense. It causes the running back to bounce outside. And he's on his own, because I have eliminated the blockers. It's one back against two or three defenders if the play has worked effectively.

Some coaches will tell you to go shoulder-to-shoulder with the lead blocker, instead of hitting him in the thigh. But sometimes that prevents you from getting both blockers.

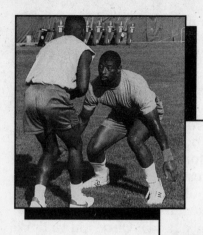

It is unsportsmanlike and dangerous to go for a player's knees.

If you have the opportunity to go for the lead blocker's thigh, make sure you have your head up. If you can get him at the waist, it's just as good. The reason you want to go for the waist or the thigh is that, in most cases, those big guys can't get that low. If they do get that low, then they're almost on the ground and they mess up the play for you. If they have to get that low to the ground, they almost have to stop to get down there—they can't keep moving. By going low, you create a logjam that brings the play to a halt.

But don't aim for the knee or below the knee or you risk getting a blow to the head. It's very easy to catch a knee in your head that snaps your head back. That can cause a concussion or more serious injury.

I would never go for a knee. A young player should never take a shot at another player's knees. It's a cardinal sin. You're not only endangering that other player, but you're also putting yourself in danger. A classic example of that would be trying to bring down Roger Craig by going for his knees. He always runs with a very high knee motion. If you go for his knees and you miss, then his knee is going to hit you right in the head. That's not good for either party.

To go for a person's knee is a very dirty play and a very dangerous play. There are some players in the league who will take shots at your knees when you're standing still. That is considered extremely dirty and it's very cowardly. A shot to the knee in that situation is going to really do some damage. But in the game of football, you never know. That's why I stress that you must always protect yourself. Never stand still on the field. Always be aware of what's happening around you.

Sometimes, players receive knee injuries by standing around a pileup, where bodies fly around. Someone might not necessarily be going for your knees, but he might fall off or fly over a pile and hit your knee. Either dive on a pile or get out of the way. Don't stand there and watch the pile. Bodies are all over the place and sometimes you can be unlucky. You can learn all the football in the world, but if you're injured you can't play the game.

Shedding blockers is a lot like making tackles because you have to deliver the blow, not take it. That's the essence of playing defense, delivering the hit instead of absorbing it. It's also a good practice to follow if you're on offense.

When a blocker and/or ballcarrier comes at you at the snap of the ball, the first thing you must know is your defensive responsibility. On the Giants, when we use a scheme called *backer force defense*, the linebacker is the last line of defense to the outside. As the outside linebacker, I absolutely cannot allow myself to be hooked or reach-blocked. If I am, then I would get sealed off to the inside and the runner could easily scamper past me on the outside.

I can avoid that by understanding my responsibility and using the proper technique to prepare for carrying it out. Before the ball is snapped, I make sure that at least a quarter or a half of my body is to the outside of the tight end. That gives me a head start getting toward the outside, which is where I can't let the play go.

Once the ball is snapped, I try to get my hands in the proper position to stalemate the blockers. Then I have to read the play. If the offense is trying to turn the corner, I have given myself an advantage by lining up favoring that side. That makes it much harder for the blocker to seal me off. If the offense succeeds in getting outside when we're in a backer force defense, it's my fault. I do whatever I can to prevent that from happening.

We also use a *safety force defense*. In that scheme, the strong safety is responsible for anything that goes outside. As the outside linebacker, I can't let the ballcarrier get between the safety and me.

In safety force, it doesn't matter if I get hook blocked. As a matter of pride, I try not to let the blocker hook me. In safety force, I play more straight up and stay on the line of scrimmage. My area of responsibility is inside the safety, which we refer to as the nine hole. I can't let myself get sucked too far inside. If I do, the safety has to

If you are a defensive player, your first concern on many plays will not be tackling the ballcarrier, but shedding a blocker. Work hard on techniques for freeing yourself, paying careful attention to using your hands to negate the blocker's advances.

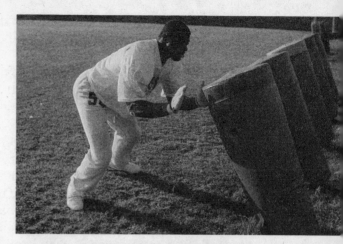

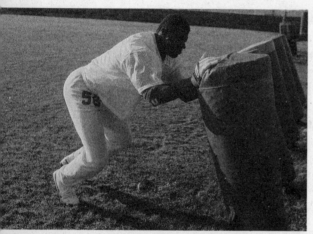

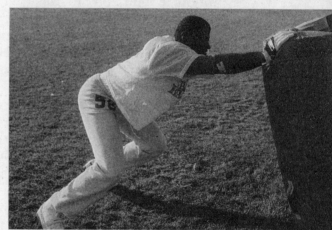

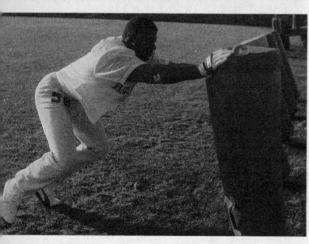

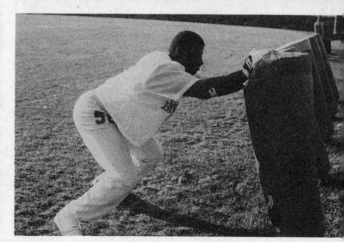

come in and fill a big void; he'll have too much space to cover between himself and the running back.

No matter what defense we're in, the key for me is to control the tight end trying to block me. I can't let him take me where he wants me to go.

I am fortunate on the Giants to have had Mark Bavaro, Zeke Mowatt, and Howard Cross as my teammates. Bavaro and Cross, of course, still butt heads with me regularly in practice. Mowatt left the Giants after the 1989 season and joined the New England Patriots.

Bavaro is very strong and an extremely hard worker. We make each other better, because we both go all out in practice. He's a great blocker and we go at each other pretty hard every day.

If he has trouble blocking me on a certain play, he'll ask me to work with him in practice on it. And if I'm having difficulty handling him on a particular play, I'll go to him. There're not a lot of secrets between us.

It's a healthy competition, because if I defeat him, he wants to know how I did it and how he can get better. I tell him and when I do, he knows what I'm going to do the next time. Then I know what he's going to do to counter it. A guy who knows you so well can help you improve, because it's talent against talent.

Mark was always an excellent blocker and he has developed into a very good receiver. After a week of practice fending off his bruising blocks, I am ready for just about anything an opposing tight end is going to try and throw at me.

As good as Bavaro is, I never had a tremendous problem shedding tight ends until 1989, when Cross joined us as a rookie out of Alabama. Howard is 6 feet 6 inches and he has unbelievably long arms. Sometimes I think he can scratch his knees without bending over.

The first day we were both in training camp, we had one-on-one drills. We went up against each other and I was surprised how well he was able to get his hands in on me. I was also dismayed that I couldn't get my hands in on him. I knew I had to attack him quickly and have very fast hands if I was going to beat Cross and any tight end like him that came along. His arms are so long that he can keep you away from his body, instead of me keeping him away from my body.

I think Howard is going to be a very good tight end. He is a good blocker primarily because of his long arms. He can knock a guy three feet off the ball because his arms are so long. I call him the stork.

I think the group of tight ends we have is the best in the league. Aside from the dynamic duo of Bavaro and Cross, I think the best pair of power-blocking tight ends in the league is in New Orleans, where Mike Tice and Hoby Brenner like to flex their muscles. Neither of these guys possesses the craftiness of an Ozzie Newsome, but that is not to downgrade their ability. They rely a great deal on strength. Both Tice and Brenner are at least 250 pounds, while Newsome is in the 235– to 240–pound range. Guys like Tice and Brenner rely on strength, and when you're playing a tight end like one of them, it's like spending your day pushing against an offensive lineman. Or an oncoming station wagon.

The battle then becomes a matter of positioning and leverage. I have to attack those big guys and attempt to neutralize them when they come off the line. Once the ball is snapped, it is a struggle to see who's going to get pushed in which direction. In order to gain some leverage, I have to be underneath their blocks. My helmet has to be beneath their helmets. If I stand straight up, I won't have any leverage, and guys like Tice and Brenner will move my body any place that suits them.

Those encounters are extremely physical and that's where conditioning comes into play. Some teams around the NFL have reputations as physical teams. These include the Washington Redskins, Chicago Bears, Saints, and, of course, the Giants. I call them power teams. When the Giants face another power team, I know I have to be in especially good condition and that my strength level must be up. That sometimes requires lifting extra weight during the course of the week, just to simulate game conditions, knowing that I'm going to be pushing a lot of weight on every play for four quarters.

If you will be lining up against an opponent who you know is more powerful and physical than most teams or players you face, make sure you do a few extra sets in the weight room during the week. Quite honestly, that is not going to give you a great difference in your strength, but it will give you an idea of how it's going to be in the game. And that extra set might give you a little additional strength, which will help you push a little longer and a little harder during a game.

During the course of an in-season workout week, you won't be able to dramatically improve your strength. But you can get accustomed to handling more weight.

The tight ends who give me the most trouble are not necessarily the strongest tight ends, but the smartest tight ends. In most cases they're veterans like Newsome. He is a very polished blocker. Newsome doesn't block with a great deal of strength, but he is what I consider a position blocker. He has a quick first step, then he might give you a quick head fake inside and then maybe jump outside on you. If you're still with him, he'll just try to ward you off. It's not a matter of strength or knocking you down, but getting in position to seal you out from the play. When I face a quick, skilled, and polished blocker like Newsome, it is imperative for me to declare my position before the ball is snapped. That may give me the edge to gain the upper hand when the play begins.

Since Newsome can jump outside in a flash, I try to line up so my inside shoulder is squared with his outside shoulder. That helps prevent me from getting sealed off by a quick blocker. By putting my body slightly to the outside of his, I will be no worse than head on with him soon after the ball is snapped. He would have to go too far outside to be able to seal me off. In a head-up position, I don't believe he will have the advantage, because he is more crafty than he is strong.

Many times during the season, I find myself in the open field with a blocker between the ballcarrier and me. It is very similar to having to make two open field tackles on one play.

The running back has many options; a lot more than if it were just the two of us in the open field. First, he knows that he has the blocker in front of him. Second, he knows that once I commit myself to taking a side on that blocker, he can go the opposite direction. Third, he will realize that if the blocker ties me up, he will have a choice of running in either direction.

Depending on the space between the ballcarrier and the blocker, you may be able to slip past the blocker and make the tackle. Keep in mind that the blocker can't be certain where the running back is behind him. It is the runner's responsibility to keep the proper distance between the two.

As a defensive player, it's very important that I get to the blocker as soon as possible, then use my hands to fend him off. There's no way in the world I can use my shoulders or forearms. If I do that,

I'm going to get tied up with the blocker. And if I spend too much time and energy ridding myself of the blocker, it will be impossible for me to make the tackle.

But by taking on the blocker with my hands, and creating separation between the two of us, I can find the running back in a hurry and make the tackle.

By now, it should be obvious to you that hand strength is very important to a football player. You can have the biggest biceps on the field, but if your hands and grip are weak, you will eventually have problems beating back those blockers and making tackles.

You can't increase your hand strength easily. Something I have done since I was young and still do today is squeeze Silly Putty. I make sure to squeeze it for the same amount of time with each hand. It's really not that strenuous. You can put a ball of putty in each hand and squeeze while you're watching television or reading. Before you know it, you'll be doing it for 30 minutes to an hour and not even realizing you've been doing it that long. The benefits will be enormous.

Another exercise I do to increase the strength in my hands is fingertip push-ups. They're very good for your grip and your finger strength. If you do enough fingertip push-ups, you can be certain you'll have the strength to grab an opponent's jersey and hold on to it when he tries to get away.

Whenever you lift weights, a side benefit will be improved hand strength. Just gripping the bar and holding on to it makes your hands and fingers stronger. Always remember that in order to be better than the guys who are doing the same as you are, you have to do extra. That's where these exercises come into play.

Hand pads are not necessary to most positions on a football team. They hurt you more than they help by restricting your hand movement. The pads certainly hamper your ability to catch a football. If you feel you want to use forearm or elbow pads, that's fine. But never use anything that's going to restrict your ability to do your job on the field. The only time I would recommend using a hand pad is if you're trying to protect a minor bruise. Hand pads give offensive players something else to grab on to.

TUESDAY

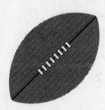

BREAKFAST: Start your day with a glass of juice. Continue with half a grapefruit or an orange, some French toast with syrup and, if you still want more fuel for your workout, eat a fruit Danish.

▼

LUNCH: Beef noodle soup with crackers, followed by baked macaroni and cheese. If you think that the latter is too heavy a dish to have before an afternoon workout, have turkey or tuna fish sandwiches on whole wheat bread instead. Don't forget to include a salad, and drink water or juice with your lunch.

▼

DINNER: For our main course tonight, we'll have a cornish hen, green beans or mixed vegetables, and dinner rolls or bread. Stick with fruit for your dessert.

Warm up.
Stretch for 30 to 40 minutes.
Run a half-mile at full speed.
Do some light stretching to prepare yourself for the sprint work you are about to do.
Run twenty 20-yard sprints. These will simulate the short distances and help you develop the short bursts of speed you need on the football field. Don't walk in between these sprints. Run 20 yards, turn around, and run your next 20 yards. After you have run each of the ten sprints, walk back to the starting line. Then run ten more sprints consecutively.
A long series of short sprints can be difficult to complete. Discipline yourself to do all twenty, to go the full 20 yards and to go hard even over the final 5 yards of your last two or three sprints. And don't start increasing the walk between sprints. Get into a good groove and don't interrupt it.
Drink fluids at regular intervals.
Jog a half-mile, carrying a football.
Stretch.
Do 30 minutes of football-related exercises.

WEDNESDAY

BREAKFAST: Start your workout day with a glass of juice and some fruit cocktail. Then have bowl of cold cereal, followed by waffles and syrup.

▼

LUNCH: This afternoon, we'll have spaghetti and meat sauce, along with a tossed salad and rolls. Drink fluid-replacement beverages with your lunch. If you want dessert, eat a bowl of sherbet or Jell-O.

▼

DINNER: Let's have one of my favorite fish dishes, swordfish. We'll have that with rice and lima beans and/or corn. Don't slip up and drink soda with your dinner. For dessert, have a bowl of ice milk and fruit. If you really want to treat yourself, put some hot fudge on it. Hey, we all deserve it. We've been working hard.

Weigh yourself before working out.
Warm up, including 5 to 10 minutes of jumping rope.
Stretch for 30 to 40 minutes.
Run two half-miles at three-quarter speed. Rest for about 3 minutes between the half-mile runs.
Drink fluids at regular intervals.
Stretch.
Do 45 minutes of football work. Start out by doing general exercises, then focus on the drills that pertain to your position.
Stretch.
Do your weight work.
Finish with 30 sit-ups and 30 push-ups.
Weigh yourself and replace fluids as needed.

You have probably noticed that we're doing more than we did last week, but not quite as much as we did in Week 6. This is because we don't want to burn out. We have reached a good level of conditioning and our job now is to maintain that conditioning. But we have stopped a step short of peak condition.

There are things you won't be able to accomplish in these personal workouts. Those are the final touches to your conditioning, which you will be able to get only in pre-season practice. That's the conditioning that comes with repetitions in practice.

You need to have something left for pre-season practice because it is going to be demanding. Since you have prepared with this program, you will be able to demand a lot of yourself. But once your body starts taking the pounding that is a big part of pre-season workouts, you will need to have something in reserve. You need room to reach that final level of conditioning.

Right now, we're maintaining the great condition that we're in. We're leaving a little room for improvement, because we're going to need it in pre-season practice.

THURSDAY

BREAKFAST: Kick off the day with juice, then have a half of honeydew melon. We'll follow that with a couple of scrambled eggs and hash brown potatoes. Eat a bagel, muffin, or piece of toast with that and have some honey.

▼

LUNCH: We'll have a good workout lunch today: a turkey club sandwich and some egg noodles. If you'd rather eat potato salad than egg noodles, go right ahead. Make sure you eat a salad and drink water or juice. If you want dessert, try a new flavor of Jell-O.

▼

DINNER: Let's get some reserve carbohydrates in our tank with manicotti and rice, our carbo special. Have carrots and/or corn with that, plus bread or rolls. Feel free to eat another salad. For dessert, try low-fat or no-fat frozen yogurt. It tastes great.

Weigh yourself before working out.
Warm up, including 5 to 10 minutes of jumping rope.

Stretch for 30 to 40 minutes.

Run a half-mile at full speed.

Do five 110-yard runs at full speed. Walk back to the starting line between sprints, then go again. Don't delay after you've reached the starting line.

Do five 50-yard sprints. Walk back to the starting line, then begin another sprint immediately.

Do five 20-yard sprints. No walking here. Do the 20-yard sprints back-to-back.

Drink fluids regularly.

Run a lap at three-quarter speed, carrying a football. Don't drop it.

Finish warming down, and stretch lightly.

Do 30 minutes of football work.

Stretch.

Weigh yourself and drink fluids to replace lost weight.

Get plenty of rest.

FRIDAY

BREAKFAST: Open up with a glass of juice, plus a grapefruit or melon half. For an alternative, try apricots. Move on to a bowl of healthful hot cereal, plus French toast with syrup or honey.

▼

LUNCH: A bowl of chicken soup or clam chowder with crackers to start. Then have cheese ravioli with cauliflower. Make sure you have a mixed green salad, and drink water or juice with your meal.

▼

DINNER: You had a good workout week, so treat yourself to pizza. You can pick your favorite toppings, but I urge you not to go too heavy on the meats. Have a salad with your dinner (I want to make sure you're getting your vegetables). Stay away from soda and other sweets. For dessert, eat your favorite fruit.

Weigh yourself before working out.

Warm up, including 10 minutes of jumping rope.

Stretch for 30 to 40 minutes.

Run a quarter-mile at full speed.

Stretch for about 10 minutes to prepare for the shorter running you are about to do.

Do four 300-yard shuttle runs.

Do four 200-yard shuttle runs.

Drink fluid-replacement beverages regularly.

Stretch lightly again.

Do 20 minutes of football work.

Do your weight work.

Finish with 30 sit-ups and 30 push-ups. Remember to work on developing your hand strength.

THE WEEKEND

 Warm up, stretch, and soak. In your spare time, work on some football exercises and agility drills. Try to do some light running. You want to keep your conditioning edge.

Continue to eat well and drink fluid-replacement beverages. Get plenty of rest.

Pre-season practice is just around the corner.

WEEK 9

This week we begin fine-tuning your body for your team's pre-season practices. Most of the pre-season hard work is finished. You should be enjoying the great condition that you're in. Right now you should be doing the little extras to make sure there is no stone left unturned.

One of the things I want you to do this week is to begin acclimating yourself to Astroturf, if you have access to an artificial turf field. If you're going to be playing games or practicing on turf, now is the time to get used to its different feel.

You don't have to do an entire workout on artificial turf, nor do you need to do anything that is very strenuous. The idea is to get accustomed to it, to get your muscles, joints, ligaments used to the preciseness of Astroturf.

Artificial turf is a completely different surface from the track or grass field you've been running on. It's very easy to pull a muscle on turf if you haven't been on it for a while. That was the problem I had during the 1988 season. I missed pre-season practice because of lengthy contract negotiations with the Giants. During that time, I worked out only on grass, an off-season mistake I will never repeat.

Turf doesn't give like grass. It's what I call very grippy. It grips your football shoes unlike the way real grass does. Your traction is much more precise on turf than it is on grass.

The feeling that I had my first day back on turf was that my muscles had tightened up, because I went right to work at full speed. Hours after I signed my contract, I practiced on the turf at Giants Stadium and I strained a muscle in my groin. I thought I had stretched well enough, but I should have been on turf earlier. There really was no time for me to ease into an artificial turf workout, to be comfortable on it before going full speed. In an ordinary situation, I would have been able to give myself a day or two just to get accustomed to the turf. I had to get right on it and my muscles tightened up because they were responding a split-second faster than they would on grass, because of the grip and the traction on turf.

Before you begin working on the turf, make sure you stretch very well. The first day you work out on the turf, just run around and get used to the field. Be alert for developing blisters, which can be just as bad as a muscle strain. Artificial turf can also be stressful on joints, which can result in weakened ankles or knees. That is another reason weight training is so important. It strengthens your joints for the pounding they will take on artificial turf.

Run around and play catch with a friend or teammate. Throw and make a few cuts on the turf, though not at full speed. Try to do an exercise that is relative to your position or positions, such as dropping back and throwing a ball or firing out of a three-point stance to get into a block. If you're a running back, jog with the football and make some light cuts. Linebackers and defensive backs should take a few pass drops.

Remember, don't go full speed your first two or three times on the turf. You just want to get your joints, ankles, and knees used to the feel of running on artificial turf. You want to see how your body responds.

There is a continuing controversy in football circles on whether playing on artificial turf causes more injuries than playing on natural grass. I honestly don't know the answer to that question. I will say that the severity of injuries sustained on artificial turf may be worse than those suffered on grass.

Grass gives more than Astroturf. If your foot is planted in natural grass, and an opponent hits your knee, the grass may come loose, saving you from a severe knee injury. But if that happens on artificial turf, the turf won't give. Your knee or ankle or whatever part of your body is going to be hit will give. But if you practice on turf, you can see how your body reacts and prepare yourself for a potentially dangerous situation.

If you fall on Astroturf, you're almost guaranteed to get a carpet burn or some kind of scratch. You really have to take care of your body when you play a number of games on turf. It puts strain on the joints, and there are problems with different injuries to the ankles or the legs or knees or something of that nature. It would be wise to ice down after a game on turf, if you're suffering problems with your knees or ankles.

MONDAY

BREAKFAST: Begin the day with a glass of your favorite juice, plus a grapefruit half or orange. Then we'll have two scrambled eggs with grits or potatoes, plus an English muffin or toast with honey. Have a ham slice or two, if you'd like.

▼

LUNCH: We'll eat a bowl of chicken soup with rice or noodles and crackers. Along with that, eat one or two turkey sandwiches on whole wheat bread. Make sure you have a tossed salad and drink water or juice. If you'd like dessert, stick with Jell-O or fruit.

▼

DINNER: Since it's our first big day of the week, we want to have an extra-good workout dinner. We'll have broiled scallops with a baked potato, peas, a salad, and dinner rolls or bread. For dessert, eat plums or peaches.

Weigh yourself before going to your workout.
Warm up, including 10 minutes of jumping rope.
Stretch for 30 to 40 minutes.
Run one or two laps at three-quarter speed to further warm your muscles for sprint work.
Stretch lightly to prepare yourself for sprint work.
Do ten 110-yard runs, walking back to the starting line between

sprints. If you are a quarterback, running back, wide receiver, defensive back, or linebacker, run these 110s holding a football.

Take a brief rest to catch your breath, then do five 60-yard sprints, with a football. No walking allowed.

Do ten 10-yard starts.

Warm down and stretch lightly.

Do 20 minutes of football exercises. The first 10 minutes should be broad-based. In the second 10 minutes, concentrate on the exercises and drills that are most relevant to your position.

After you have finished your football exercises, stretch, taking extra care if you have been working on artificial turf.

Do your weight work.

Finish with 30 sit-ups and 30 push-ups.

Weigh yourself and replace lost fluids.

If you are a defensive lineman, you should be working on your pass-rushing moves. Rushing the passer may look like one of the simplest, most basic skills in football: the quarterback drops back, and the defensive linemen try to bull their way past their offensive counterparts to disengage the quarterback from the ball. In some respects, it is little more than that.

But contrary to what it may look like to the average fan or the young player, rushing the passer requires a lot of technique and a lot of thought. It takes just as much responsibility to rush the passer as it does to cover a receiver or bring down a runner on the loose.

Pressuring the quarterback is a vital part of defensive football, particularly on third down. The best play you can get in a situation like that is a quarterback sack.

But you don't just leave it to chance. Every team has several plays designed for getting to the quarterback. The essential point to remember about rushing the passer is that you want to get the man blocking you to go one way while you go the other. If you don't think it's easier to do it that way, try running into a strong, 300-pound guy every down, pushing him straight back into the quarterback. Pretty soon, you'll be looking for a place to lie down.

I have had the pleasure of playing with the man who is, in my opinion, the master of the pass rush, Lawrence Taylor. Just watching him everyday in practices and games has made me a much better pass rusher. He is a perfectionist when it comes to sacking the quarterback.

The first object of a pass rusher is to trick the offensive lineman trying to block him. The problem is that most of those guys are pretty smart, so they don't go for every fake that you have. To combat that, you have to have a systematic way of going about your job. You need a countermove for every counter that he has for your first move. So you have to counter his counter at times. Got it?

The basic pass rush move is what we call the *slap uppercut*. You take three steps in one direction, drive a hard head fake in that direction, then slap the blocker's shoulder or another part of his upper body, with the opposite hand, upper cut, and you go around him. Many youth football leagues don't allow hand slapping. If yours does not, you will have to rely more on your faking ability and strength to get to the quarterback. If you are not allowed to use your hands, go three steps one way and give the blocker a good head fake, then go back the other way.

You can also try a *spin move*. Step forward until you are directly in front of the blocker. Give him a quick fake one way, then spin all the way around and past him. If it works, you will have a clear path to the quarterback.

The key to pass rushing, as with so many facets of playing defensive football, is knowing what your responsibility is. Where do you have to be? Are you the outside rusher or the inside rusher?

It's a lot like playing the run or pass when you are a linebacker. If you are the outside rusher, then you know you can't get caught inside. Being the outside rusher means you are the contain man. If you are responsible for containing the quarterback, you can't let him get outside the passing pocket; you have to contain him inside. If he gets outside and runs for a long gain, the breakdown is your fault. With that responsibility, you can make all the moves you want as long as your last move is to the outside. The quarterback has to stay inside of you.

If you are the outside rusher, sometimes a big hole will open up toward the inside. You may think you can get through it, but as soon as you get there, the offensive lineman will wall you off so you can't get back outside. The quarterback will step outside of the pocket, where he can bide more time and release the pass, or run down the field and gain the yardage himself. Even if it is tempting to try another route, you must do what your responsibility on that play demands. Don't try to free-lance, unless you are 100 percent certain you can get there.

The only time I would consider gambling is when we're facing a quarterback who is not mobile and whose scrambling ability is limited. Neil Lomax, who used to play for the Phoenix Cardinals, comes to mind, though you had to be careful against him because he was such a good passer. With a classic pocket quarterback like Lomax, every once in a while you can get away with an inside move. You have to make sure you make the move deep enough. If it's done too close to the line of scrimmage, even a plodder like Lomax can get around you. You have to go upfield far enough and then make your move underneath. A pocket passer like Lomax will get to a certain point in his drop-back, then step up to release the ball. If you're fortunate, an inside move will leave you at the same spot at the same time.

I have to be even more mobile playing against a quarterback such as Randall Cunningham, who is so elusive. If I go the wrong way while rushing Randall, he can easily step aside or around me and damage a defense by himself.

When rushing any quarterback, especially one as adept as Cunningham, the most important rule to follow is to stay on your feet. He is a great pump faker with a long release. He looks like he's about to let the ball go, but at the last moment, just before he is about to release it, he somehow brings it back. In a game in the Meadowlands in 1987, he fooled me three times that way. I was certain he was going to throw it and I jumped. While I was in the air, he would run past me or head to safer territory until he found an open receiver.

My high school basketball coach used to say, "Don't jump unless you have a parachute." That sequence was also embarrassing and though it wasn't as striking as the missed tackle in Philadelphia that I described earlier, it's something that a lot of people remember.

I learned my lesson that year. When we played them again three weeks later, I sacked Cunningham three times. That didn't seem to get nearly the same amount of attention my gaffes did, but it was satisfying for me to know that I had improved from one game to the next.

You have to be tentative at times when you're rushing Cunningham. We like to try and trap him and give him just one place to go, to limit his options in any given play. One of Cunningham's overlooked attributes is that he's a quick thinker. He thinks well on the run.

Cunningham is such a difficult quarterback to prepare for because there are so many factors to his football game. He's an extremely good runner, great improviser, and has a very strong arm. With that combination in one player, it makes it difficult to prepare for. What do you tell your defense? Be ready for everything?

I think the key to stopping Randall Cunningham is to control his ten teammates on the field as best as you can, because no matter how good he is, he can't do it all himself. You have to get to Cunningham when you can, but if you can shut down the rest of the Eagles' offense, you'll be all right. I'm not saying that he's not capable of winning games singlehandedly, but in the game of football, that's very rare. You can have a couple of games here and there where one player really turns it around and wins it for you. But it's almost impossible for one player to keep a team on top throughout a season.

If the talent levels of their teams are equal, I would prefer to play a straight drop-back quarterback such as Jim Everett of the Rams than someone like Cunningham, who can also hurt your game by running. But with the offensive line and receivers that Everett has, he can be very tough. He proved that to us in both the 1988 and 1989 seasons.

Everett threw for five touchdowns against us at Giants Stadium on September 25, 1988, and the Rams beat us handily, 45–31. We played them again in Anaheim on November 12, 1989. That time, Everett threw for 295 yards and two touchdowns, and we lost, 31–10.

I think Everett is most accurate when he's in the pocket and not on the run. When he's moving, he doesn't throw with the same accuracy as he does when he's standing in the pocket, because he's not used to moving around. If Everett scrambles to avoid a sack, he normally has to set his feet again before throwing the ball. That is quite a difference from John Elway or Cunningham, because they can throw on a dead run with very good accuracy.

If you have containment responsibilities on a pocket passer, there's a good chance you won't get the sack running straight up the field at the quarterback. I try to rush the quarterback from one side, about a yard deeper than he sets up. I then make my move to the inside. You can't just go to the same level as the quarterback, because he'll know there's a pocket collapsing around him and he'll step out to make a pass.

Pocket quarterbacks are now taking shorter pass drops than they used to. If you play against a quarterback who is taking short drops, then you are going to have to shorten your pass rush. If the offensive team has a solid wall in front for the inside guys, it is very difficult to get a good angle on the quarterback. With a quarterback who takes a short drop, you really have to depend on the interior guys to put pressure on the quarterback. That should force him to go deeper than he wants to.

With quarterbacks who are more mobile you simply don't take a chance, because they can burn you. Elway and Cunningham are extremely effective throwing or running if they get time and room to move around, so it is imperative to keep them in the pocket.

The same is true of Joe Montana. They are the kinds of quarterbacks who have to be contained at all costs. The way to do that is by rushing them from the outside in. An inside rush is an invitation to those quarterbacks to do what they want. They'll have time to move away from the rush and to make time until they find an open receiver.

In the Giants' defensive scheme, the outside linebacker is most often an outside pass rusher. That means, of course, that I have contain responsibility on the quarterback. There are instances where we have different pass rush games or stunts, which allow me to be an inside rusher or to make a free move. A free move enables me to go wherever I want, because one of my teammates is going to be rushing outside of me. That teammate will take over the contain responsibility.

The ideal situation for a rushing outside linebacker is to be one-on-one with a back. Since a back is usually shorter and weaker than a linebacker, the defensive player should have the advantage in that matchup. But that very seldom happens.

We try to create situations where we are rushing the passer from the side where the back is going out for a pass pattern, and the offensive tackle is blocking the defensive end. That should leave you as a pass rusher without a blocker to pick you up.

Unfortunately for me, that doesn't happen too frequently during the course of a season. Most often, I have a huge tackle right in front of me, blocking my path to the quarterback. The toughest I face is Joe Jacoby of the Redskins, who is 6 feet 7 inches tall and at least 305 pounds. He is so wide you can't go around him and so big you can't go through him. You have to use some technique and try to get him to go in one direction while you go the opposite way. The problem with facing Jacoby is that his arms are so long, you really have to sell this guy with your fake. All he has to do to slow you down is get one arm on you. I'm at a little bit of a disadvantage

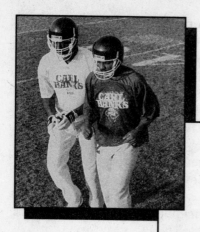

If you are the outside pass rusher, you must contain the quarterback.

when we play, because I don't rush the passer as often as LT, who is very familiar with Jacoby's moves. But this is an example of how I can watch Taylor and incorporate what I've learned into my own game.

Luis Sharpe gives me problems on pass rushes for another reason. He's not as big as Jacoby, but he's a very, very talented athlete and he's very smart. Many times, it seems that Sharpe has an answer for every move I make. He knows what to do with almost every trick I have.

There are different things you can try during a game to get around a blocker and sack the quarterback. There's the slap uppercut, a spin move, a slap/grab uppercut, and a double slap. But before you can use any of these, you must get the basic fakes and footwork down.

If you have the outside rush, you must, by all means, stay outside of the tackle. Under no circumstances can you let him drive you inside. You have to make a good move that not only advances you toward the quarterback, but keeps you outside. The key there is to really sell the blocker on your inside fake. If you're an outside rusher and you want to be a part of the sack, instead of just acting as a diversion for the tackle, you have to make a good inside fake and get back outside in enough time to make the tackle.

Let's assume you have convinced the blocker to go for your inside fake; you have stepped outside and you now have a clear path to the quarterback. It's a great situation to be in, but your job is far from through. That quarterback might be very elusive, so you may have to outwit him before you sack him.

As I mentioned earlier, you don't want to go in and try to block the pass, though your natural instincts may tell you to jump up and try to bat the pass down. If you decide you want to try and block the throw, don't leave your feet. If you do, the quarterback will step around you, where he can complete his pass or start running upfield. Most of the time, it's the second or third rusher who bats the ball down.

If you have time, you want to make the tackle. And to be honest, most quarterbacks don't have time to think about how they're going to avoid you. When they are sitting in the pocket, all they want to do is get rid of the ball or get out of the way.

When you are bearing down on a quarterback, it's best to look at his waist, just as you do when a running back is bearing down on you in the open field. You will be much less susceptible to a fake if you have your eyes focused on his waist. In the 1987 season, I made a move and found myself with a clear path to Dallas quarterback Danny White. I broke his wrist on the play, which I didn't mean to do, of course. He tried to step up in the pocket, but since I was concentrating on his waist, he could do nothing to fool me.

TUESDAY

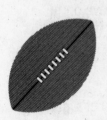

BREAKFAST: Kick off with a glass of juice, plus a half of cantaloupe. Have a healthful bowl of hot or cold cereal, taking care to avoid those with a high sugar content. Have a muffin, bagel, or toast with your cereal, plus a cup of low-fat yogurt.

▼

LUNCH: Have a bowl of vegetable or lentil soup with crackers. Along with that, have one or two grilled ham-and-cheese sandwiches. But not just any ham and cheese. Use boiled ham, low-fat cheese, and margarine instead of butter. Include a mixed green salad, and drink water or juice with your meal. If you feel like dessert, try some sherbet.

DINNER: Our main course tonight will be baked or barbecued chicken, whichever you prefer. We'll have lima beans and corn with that, plus mashed potatoes (use margarine, not sour cream or butter). Don't drink soda with your meal. For dessert, eat a banana or two.

Warm up, including 10 minutes of jumping rope.

Stretch for 30 to 40 minutes.

Run a half-mile at three-quarter speed, carrying a football.

Do four 220-yard runs at full speed. Jog back to the starting lineup between runs. Catch your breath if necessary, but don't dawdle before starting over. Make sure you go all out all the way. Don't let up in the last 10 or 20 yards.

Stretch lightly for 5 or 10 minutes.

Do four 150-yard shuttle runs with a football. Time yourself. See if you can finish each one in 25 to 30 seconds, which, at this stage of the program, shouldn't be difficult. Don't take more than 30 seconds between shuttle runs.

Drink fluids throughout your workout.

Warm down and stretch.

WEDNESDAY

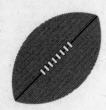

BREAKFAST: Begin the day with your favorite juice. Then move on to a stack of pancakes, either plain, apple, or blueberry, with syrup. If there's room, have a fruit Danish.

▼

LUNCH: Start with a bowl of navy bean soup and crackers. Let's get some extra carbohydrates today and eat spaghetti with tomato or marinara sauce. Make sure you have both a green salad and your fluid-replacement beverages.

▼

DINNER: Tonight we'll enjoy roast pork loin with applesauce. With that, eat string beans and red potatoes, plus rolls or bread. Drink water or juice with your meal. Finish your meal with red or green grapes.

Check your weight before leaving the house.
Warm up, including 10 minutes of jumping rope.
Stretch for 30 to 40 minutes.
Run one lap around the football field at three-quarter speed.
Do five 220-yard runs at full speed. Jog back to the starting lineup between runs. As you did yesterday, catch your breath so you can continue to run at full speed, but don't take an unnecessarily long break between runs. Go all out on every sprint. Don't pull up until you have run the complete 220 yards.
Do five 100-yard full strides on the football field. Striding is running at three-quarter speed. It is not a sprint. These should be done carrying a football.
Drink fluid-replacement drinks throughout your workout.
Warm down and stretch.
Do 20 minutes of football exercises, starting on those that are more general and moving on to those used in your position or positions.
Do your weight work.
Finish with 30 sit-ups and 30 push-ups.

THURSDAY

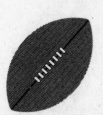

BREAKFAST: Begin your day with a glass of juice. Today we'll have a fruit cocktail with low-fat yogurt, an English muffin with honey, and French toast with syrup.

▼

LUNCH: Today, we'll have a bowl of pea soup with crackers. Then you have a choice. For those of you with larger appetites, have macaroni and cheese. If you'd rather not eat that much, have a turkey or chicken sandwich on whole wheat bread. No matter what you choose, eat a salad and drink fluid-replacement beverages.

▼

DINNER: Tonight we'll enjoy baked cod, flounder, or halibut. Don't use tartar sauce, because it has too much fat. Use lemon to flavor your fish. We'll have broccoli and cauliflower with that and be sure to eat dinner rolls or bread. For dessert, have a piece or two of your favorite fruit.

Warm up, including 10 minutes of jumping rope.

Stretch for 30 to 40 minutes. Since you are nearing the end of your ninth workout week, you may think you can cut this to 20 or even 10 minutes. Get that thought out of your head right now. Even if you've been stretching every day for a year, you shouldn't cut short your stretching time.

By now you should be getting far down on your stretches, much further than you could three or four weeks ago and much, much further than when we began. But that doesn't mean your muscles are stretched permanently, nor is it a sign that you can't improve. You have to keep putting in your time stretching each day, to keep your body limber and to continue building on what you've started.

Run two laps around the field carrying a football.

Run five 100-yard sprints full speed on the field. Don't rest for more than a minute between sprints.

When you're finished with your 100-yard sprints, take a rest of no longer than 5 minutes and drink fluids. Then run five 80-yard sprints on the field.

Take another brief rest and run five 60-yard sprints on the field.

Follow those with five 20-yard sprints.

Walk once around the field to warm down. Drink fluids as needed. Be careful not to drink so much that you get bloated. We're not finished yet.

Stretch lightly for 5 minutes.

Run five 40-yard sprints. Go hard and don't let up until you have run the full 40 yards. Catch your breath between sprints, but don't stand around and admire the sunshine.

Take another brief break, then run ten 10-yard starts. If you play a position that requires you to get down in a three-point stance, then do these starts from that football position.

Stretch and warm down.

Finish with 30 sit-ups and 30 push-ups.
Drink fluids to replace lost weight.

FRIDAY

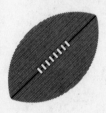

BREAKFAST: Begin the day with a glass of juice, then have some pear halves or honeydew melon. Follow that up with a bowl or two of healthful hot or cold cereal (or one of each if you'd like), plus a muffin, bagel, or toast with honey.

▼

LUNCH: I want you to eat pasta today, so have lasagna, spaghetti, or ravioli as your main course. Eat green beans with that, as well as a mixed green salad. Make sure you are still putting low-fat dressing on your salad. Drink water, juice, or low-fat milk with your lunch.

▼

DINNER: You've earned a Friday reward this week, so have prime ribs of beef for dinner. Make sure it's lean, of course, and get rid of as much fat as you can. Have broccoli and a baked potato with that, as well as a salad. Drink water, juice, or low-fat milk with your meal. For dessert, eat ice milk or low-fat frozen yogurt.

Try to get a partner for today's workout. We'll be doing a lot of football exercises and drills and you will be able to accomplish much more if you have someone else to participate with.

Weigh yourself before working out.

Warm up, including 10 minutes of jumping rope.

Stretch for 30 to 40 minutes.

Run goal post to goal post at three-quarter speed with the ball.

Run five 60-yard sprints.

Run ten 20-yard sprints.

Do 1 hour of football work. Just because you're not sprinting, don't slack off. Work hard. For everyone except quarterbacks, make sure you get in your tire work and bag work.

When you are done, jog two laps around the field.
Drink fluids throughout the workout.
Stretch to prepare for lifting weights.
Do your weight work.
Finish with 30 sit-ups and 30 push-ups.

THE WEEKEND

Maintain your good dietary habits. Each day, you should warm up, stretch, and soak. Since we are so close to the beginning of your team's pre-season workouts, you should also do at least a half-hour of football exercises each day. This will put you at an advantage when practice begins. Many of your teammates may be a little uncomfortable doing football exercises early in camp. They won't be able to do them at full speed, because they will not have practiced them before arriving at camp.

But you will be able to go all out from day one. It's the time and effort you put in now that will give you an edge when practice starts and throughout the season. I know that many of the big plays I make during the year are due to the sacrifices I make in this program.

On December 16, 1989, the Giants played the Dallas Cowboys in the Meadowlands. The game was close, and late in the third period the Cowboys were right on our doorstep with a first and goal.

We stopped them on three consecutive plays. On fourth down, they ran a sweep to their offensive left for Paul Palmer, an unusual play in a goal line situation, because it takes so long to develop.

I was playing on the opposite side, our defensive left, their offensive right. Because they wanted big bodies down near the goal line, they removed their tight end and stacked their front wall with huge offensive linemen.

I knew that if they were going to run the ball my way, I was going to have to stay low. I would probably just bury myself in the ground, so I wouldn't get pushed off the ball. But I've learned something about offensive linemen. When the play is not going their way, they tend to relax a little bit. That's what the man opposite me did. When I saw him relax, I figured the play was going to the other side.

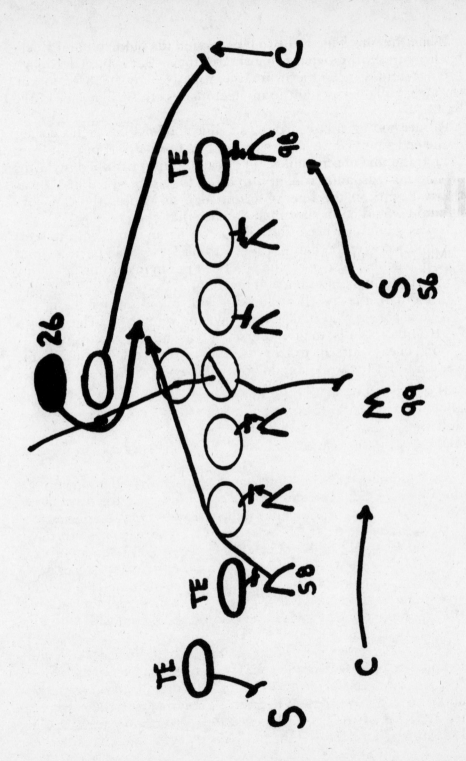

I stopped this fourth down attempt by the Dallas Cowboys to score against us at Giants Stadium late in the 1989 season. Paul Palmer ran a sweep to our defensive right side. I took off from the left side and tackled Palmer for a 3-yard loss, the Cowboys' last chance to score in a game we won, 15–0.

When the play began, the Cowboys tried to cut me off and shield me from running down the line of scrimmage. But I slipped through a crack and saw Palmer with the ball. He had no hole to run through, which is a credit to my teammates on the play side of the ball.

Palmer had to run toward the sideline and hope to catch a corner of the end zone. While he was doing that, I was in hot pursuit from behind the line of scrimmage and I caught him, wrapped my arms around his legs, and brought him down for a three-yard loss. I was the last man on the line of scrimmage, so I guess the Cowboys figured I would be the last man to make that play.

It was a big play, because Dallas never again came close to scoring, and we won the game, 15–0. I think I was able to make that play, in part, because of all the practice I put in in coming out of my stance, changing direction, and tackling.

In football, they're all basic skills. But if you master them, you can be a player who makes big plays for your team. The time to work on those skills, to give yourself a season-long edge, is now.

Don't cheat yourself. You may want to take a break because it's the weekend. But the work you do now will pay off during the season.

WEEK 10

Congratulations. You are about to cross the finish line of your own workout program. Soon you will be at the mercy of your coaches. But if you have prepared well and followed this program, the fatigue you see on the faces of others won't be experienced by you.

By now you should be in pretty darn good shape. You understand what it takes to get into shape. With pre-season practice just around the corner, there's no need to overdo it and risk pulling a muscle or suffering some other debilitating injury. Right now all you need to do is maintain your condition and make sure you are peaking as you go into pre-season practice.

When you get there, you should be one of the guys the coaches refer to as somebody who did a lot of work during the off-season. You should be the positive example for the players who are bent over and have their heads in a trash can, who can't keep up because they spent their summer sitting around, conserving their energy.

This is the point at which all your dreams become realizations. You've worked hard to prepare yourself for a grueling season. Now you are ready for the pre-season workout. When the going gets tough—as it inevitably does in every football season—you'll know that you have what it takes to keep going and reach the goals you've worked so hard to achieve during the summer.

You have prepared yourself mentally and physically. Pre-season practice is never easy. But if you have done your work, it will be easier for you than it will be for a lot of other guys in the league and on your team. You should now feel that your body is strong enough to enable you to excel through twice-a-day practices.

Pre-season practice is the time coaches use to see that their players are in shape and to make sure they can get things down mentally before the regular season begins. Now that you are prepared physically, you will also be a lot sharper mentally. You've been working hard for ten weeks. You will feel the benefits from that when pre-season workouts begin.

Most coaches assume their players are out of shape, so they design their practices to be very demanding. They won't seem as difficult to you as they do to your teammates if you show up in excellent shape.

We will not run as much as we have in recent weeks. And you should taper off your weight work this week. Work lightly, including decreasing the weight in some of your exercises if a part of your body feels weary. It is important that you be well rested for pre-season practice.

By the tenth week, if you're not where you want to be with the weights, there's no sense in trying to get there now. If you haven't reached your goals in nine weeks, you won't make a drastic improvement now. It has to be a gradual change.

Your work, of course, is really just beginning. But by completing this program, you have given yourself a big head start.

MONDAY

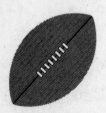

BREAKFAST: Start with a glass of juice and a bowl of strawberries or blueberries (or mix them up). Then have two or three scrambled eggs with potatoes or grits, and a muffin, bagel, or toast with honey.

▼

LUNCH: We'll open up with a bowl of vegetable soup with crackers, followed by stuffed pasta shells, peas, and a mixed green salad. Drink water or fruit juice with your meal. Eat an apple for dessert.

▼

DINNER: Pick your favorite fish dish, such as scrod, cod, halibut, or swordfish, and have it baked or grilled—not fried. If you require additional flavoring, use lemon juice or cocktail sauce. Have some hot mixed vegetables with that, as well a rice dish and dinner rolls. For dessert, eat peaches, plums, or nectarines.

Weigh yourself before working out. You should be at or extremely close to your pre-season practice reporting weight, set either by you or your coaches.

Warm up, including 10 minutes of jumping rope.

Stretch for 30 to 40 minutes. Don't rush through your stretches because it's the last week of the program. Stretching is even more important now, because pre-season practice is so close. A muscle pull now may jeopardize your chance to make the team or cost you a lot of playing time. If anything, you should be doing extra stretching this week.

Jog two laps around the football field, just enough to break a sweat.

Do four 100-yard runs, striding. By now you should know that striding does not mean a full-speed, all-out sprint. At the same time, it doesn't mean you should take a lazy stroll from one end of the field to the other. This is not a demanding exercise, but that doesn't mean you should do it without effort.

Do 30 minutes of football work, concentrating the final 15 minutes on those that are most suited to your position.

Drink fluids throughout the workout.

Stretch for about 10 minutes.

Do some light weight work, enough to keep your conditioning edge. Sit-ups and push-ups are optional, though recommended.

TUESDAY

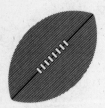

BREAKFAST: We'll begin today with a glass of juice and a grapefruit half, orange, or tangerine. Then eat plain or fruit pancakes with syrup or honey, plus a fruit Danish or muffin if you have room.

▼

LUNCH: Chicken soup with rice or noodles, along with a tuna fish, chicken salad, or seafood sandwich or two. Eat a hot vegetable, such as green beans or corn with that, as well as your salad. Drink water or juice and complete the meal with a bowl of Jell-O.

▼

DINNER: Our main dish this evening will be barbecued, baked, or broiled chicken, along with mashed potatoes, broccoli, and cauliflower, and rolls or cornbread. For dessert, treat yourself to a piece of fruit pie, such as apple, cherry, or blueberry.

Weigh yourself before going to your workout.

Warm up and stretch for 1 hour. Yes, a full hour. I want you stretched and limber for the beginning of pre-season practice.

It is very, very important that you continue to stretch during the course of the season, especially when the weather turns cold. It is much harder to stretch muscles when they are cold. In cold weather, you are very susceptible to pulls. The coaches are demanding we give 100 percent effort in practice, so we can complete our offensive and defensive preparations and get our timing down.

We all stretch at the beginning of practice, but that primarily benefits the players who practice first. On the Giants, the offensive and defensive units alternate practicing first. If the offense goes first, then I could stand around for 45 minutes. When it's time for me to go with the rest of the defense, I have to be loose. The way to do that is to keep moving around and keep stretching. If you just stand around when it's cold outside, your muscles will tighten up quickly and you will be risking a pull that could send you to the sidelines.

WEDNESDAY

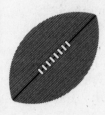

BREAKFAST: Begin your day with a glass of juice and a fruit cocktail. Follow that with a bowl of healthful cold cereal, plus waffles and syrup or honey. If you need more fuel, eat an orange or apple.

▼

LUNCH: Eat a bowl of navy bean or lentil soup with crackers, then a hot turkey or chicken sandwich with whole wheat bread. Have some carrots with that, as well as a salad. Drink water or juice and complete your lunch with a piece or two of your favorite fruit.

▼

DINNER: Tonight we'll have chicken parmigiana with spaghetti and tomato sauce on the side. We can't forget vegetables, so include some peas and/or corn with your meal. Have a bowl of ice milk with fruit for dessert.

Weigh yourself before working out.
Warm up, including 10 minutes of jumping rope.
Stretch for at least 45 minutes.
Jog two laps around the football field.
Stretch briefly.
Run two 110-yard sprints at striding speed.
Run four 60-yard sprints at close to top speed.
Run six 20-yard starts.
Drink fluids throughout your workout.
Do 30 minutes of football exercises and drills, the last 15 minutes on drills for your position.
When you have completed your football exercises, stretch.
Do some light weight work, including sit-ups and push-ups.

Despite all the time you've put into this program, and all the preparation you've made, everything is not always going to go your way. Far from it. You're going to make mistakes. You will probably come up against a player who is better than you. Your team is going to lose games.

Through all the good times and bad, the one constant in your football life should be hustle. You must never let up on the football field. A lot of mistakes can be tolerated by football players and coaches. But failure to try hard at all times is not one of them. A never-say-die competitive spirit can compensate for a lot of deficiencies and weaknesses.

I'm a strong believer that if you give 100 percent effort at all times, good fortune will find you on the football field. It found me in the second quarter of a game against the Seattle Seahawks on November 19, 1989, at Giants Stadium. I learned once again that sometimes it is better to be lucky than good.

We were leading 7–0 midway through the second period when the Seahawks faced a third-and-10 from their own 43-yard line. We were in a nickel defense (in which we use an extra defensive back) and I was supposed to be covering wide receiver Paul Skansi. He got away from me, however, and was open when quarterback Kelly Stouffer threw him a pass.

I didn't give up, and was hustling after Skansi when the pass was thrown. Despite that, it looked to be a certain completion, before fortune intervened.

The ball bounced off Skansi's hands and right into my own for my first interception of the season. I would not have gotten it if I had stopped hustling when it appeared I was hopelessly beat.

I had coverage on Skansi, but it was very poor coverage. But the ball popped out of his hands. If I hadn't been alert, or if I felt that I had been beat and didn't have to keep hustling, then the ball would have hit the ground. But I continued to chase after the receiver and the ball dropped out of his hands right into mine.

It always pays to keep hustling. That interception was the perfect example of not knowing when a play is going to be over. The play's not over till the whistle's blown. So if you're beat just keep hustling and try to get to the man with the ball. You might get an interception, or even a touchdown out of it.

THURSDAY

BREAKFAST: Start off with a glass of juice and a grapefruit half. Then have a bowl or two of healthful hot cereal, taking care to avoid those with added sugar. Finish off the meal with a muffin, bagel, or piece of toast with honey.

▼

LUNCH: Have a bowl of vegetable soup or clam chowder with crackers. Then we'll have one or two hamburgers made with very lean ground beef. If you prefer cheeseburgers, use low-fat cheese. You can have french fries, but don't fry them in oil. Heat them up by baking them. Eat your salad and drink water, juice, or low-fat milk. For dessert, sample your favorite fruit.

▼

DINNER: Tonight we'll eat a veal chop with your choice of potato and broccoli or asparagus. Remember to drink water or juice with your meal. For dessert, have ice milk or low-fat frozen yogurt.

Warm up, including 10 minutes of jumping rope.
Run a half-mile. Stride, don't sprint.
Run 110 yards 4 times. Again, do this striding.
Do 15 minutes of football exercises.

FRIDAY

BREAKFAST: Welcome to the final day of our workout program. Get off to a good start with a glass of your favorite juice and a cantaloupe or honeydew half. Then have a bowl of cold cereal, preferably corn, oat, wheat, or bran flakes. Finish up with French toast and syrup or honey.

▼

LUNCH: Start with a bowl of vegetable soup. If you want to reward yourself for reaching the end of the program, eat pizza with your choice of topping. Follow our rules, though, and go easy on the meat. If you'd rather not eat pizza, have turkey sandwiches on whole wheat bread. No matter what you choose, make sure to eat a salad. Maintain your discipline and don't drink soda. Have Jell-O or fruit for dessert.

▼

DINNER: It's the final night of the program, so treat yourself and celebrate. Enjoy a sirloin or T-bone steak or a prime rib. Whatever you choose, make sure it is lean. You're in great shape now, but that doesn't mean you should eat extra fat. With your steak, have mushrooms, broccoli, and a baked potato, plus dinner rolls and bread. For dessert, have a bowl of ice milk with strawberries or low-fat frozen yogurt.

Weigh yourself before working out. This is a good habit to maintain once you begin training, because the work will be hard and you could sweat off several pounds during a workout. You're going to have to replace that lost weight with fluid-replacement beverages.

Warm up, including 10 minutes of jumping rope.

Stretch for at least 45 minutes.

What you do the rest of the day will depend on when practice begins. Assuming it starts the following Monday, jog a mile very lightly and stride 100 yards 4 times.

Do a light football exercise for about 10 or 15 minutes, even if it's just playing catch with a friend for a few minutes.

If your practice doesn't begin until the middle of the following week, do a full 30 minutes of exercises and work hard at them. Keep stretching. Jog a lap or two. Work lightly in the weight room. Try to limit the strain on your legs, which will be taxed enough when you get to camp.

THE WEEKEND

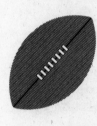

Stretch, soak, and relax. Get mentally ready for pre-season practice.

Keep in mind that you have worked hard and you are in shape, but you are still going to experience soreness when you get to practice. Don't think that you are out of shape because you're sore. When you get to practice, you will be using some muscles and doing things that have been totally different from what you have been doing the last 10 weeks. Coaches always manage to come up with a drill that will give you a sore spot where you didn't even know you had a spot. You will also be sore because of the personal contact in football.

You can get a good indication of your condition after running a play. You should be recovering after each play with plenty of time to spare. If you haven't recovered fully and you are still tired when the next play begins, then it may be wise to do a little extra running after practice.

But don't do too much. Most pre-season workouts are designed to get you tired. If you're in shape, you will know it. Mentally, you'll feel good after practice. Physically, you will be a little sore, but you should be sore.

As practice continues and your body gets a little tired or you feel a little fatigued mentally, get into a whirlpool or tub after practice. If the weather is hot, take a cold whirlpool or tub bath. You don't have to put your whole body in. It helps to revive the legs.

Finally, it is very important that you do get enough rest. You're going to need every ounce of energy for the next practice. You can't perform at your best if you are tired. And if you are fatigued, you put yourself at much greater risk of sustaining an injury. Don't short-change yourself on sleep.

During the season, maintain the good dietary habits you've developed during this program. Oh, you can splurge once in a while and eat something that's not on your menu. Just don't make a regular habit of it.

Keep working hard, and good luck in the football season. Monitoring your weight and drinking fluids regularly are habits you should take from this program and use consistently. You've given yourself an edge. Now use it.

DRUGS

All the time and effort you have spent getting into excellent condition will be wasted if you use drugs. Drugs can destroy your life. If you are fortunate enough to function semi-normally when you use drugs, there is no way you can perform your best on the football field. The best advice I could ever give you is: Stay away from drugs.

I have never taken drugs of any kind. But I have seen the lives of many other people destroyed because they used drugs. When I talk to youngsters, they ask me why haven't I ever used and why won't I ever try drugs. I make sure to tell them that drugs are no good for their bodies and are terribly unhealthy. I warn them that drugs can ruin their lives and destroy their dreams. Worse, drugs can kill you.

But I also tell them that there are a lot of people who look up to me and there are many people who are proud of me. When you are successful, your parents brag about you. They say, "That's my boy." They bring the newspaper clippings to work to show their friends. And their friends say, "I know that young man's mother. I work with her." Everybody is bragging about you and looking up to you. Naturally, you love it.

My parents were the proudest people when I succeeded at football. They were the people that I wanted to keep happy. If I was ever in the newspapers because of drugs, how could they go face their friends and everyone else they bragged to? And how could those people, who bragged about me to *their* friends, not feel embarrassed?

If you get involved with drugs, you not only humiliate yourself, but you embarrass a lot of other people. The most obvious, and the people who are going to be hurt the most, are your parents. The last thing I ever want to do is hurt my parents.

Many times when I pick up a newspaper I read that some athlete or former athlete—whether it's football, baseball, basketball, or track—has been caught using drugs or accused of using drugs. It always disappoints me a great deal, to a degree that only my closest friends know.

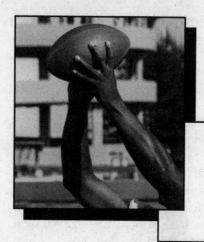

There is no way you can be in top condition if you are taking drugs. Drugs have no place in sports.

Maybe I'm a little old-fashioned. But I'm a true believer that athletes should have pure, clean bodies. I believe just as strongly that professional athletes should be the ultimate example for kids. I know that a lot of athletes don't want to be role models. But whether they like it or not, they are. As professionals, as collegians, and even as high school kids, at some level we are role models and someone is looking up to us.

Drugs have no place in sports. It really hurts to discover that someone you know, that someone you play with, is involved with drugs.

I have worked extremely hard to be a positive example for the sport that I represent. It's very disturbing to find out someone is using drugs, because I've tried so hard to keep the sport the way it should be, which is pure and clean as far as athletics is concerned. It means a great deal to me to be a positive role model for my sport and the team that I represent. If someone else is going to destroy that positive image and give kids something negative to think about in their life's choices, I think that is an injustice to someone so young and so easily influenced.

It really upsets me. The older guys sometimes forget that they were once kids. They looked up to somebody. They can say that they didn't, but I know they did. There was somebody who they liked in sports. They should realize that somebody is looking up to them, especially because they are at the professional level.

All of pro sports has taken a black eye because of a few knuckleheads. Then you get a few kids who say, "If he can do it and he is still doing well, then I can do it." I'm here to tell you that it isn't true. You will be destroying your body just like any other person who is stupid enough to take drugs. If he got caught, you will get caught also. The consequences could be devastating.

There is simply no way you can succeed when you use drugs. No one has ever made himself better by using drugs. Neither I nor anyone else has ever seen a positive example from someone who uses drugs. But a lot of players have hurt themselves in a lot of ways because of them.

If you are using drugs while you are trying to get in shape using my program, you can forget about completing it or even gaining anything from it. You won't get anything close to the maximum benefits. Every day will be spent fighting to make up what you lost because of your drug abuse. You will be trying to build your body up, but the drugs will really be tearing it down.

I understand that you may be subjected to a great deal of peer pressure to try and to use drugs. Some of your friends may use them and you may feel you will be ostracized by the group if you don't join in. In that situation, you have to be strong and hold on to your goals. Or you can be weak and fall prey to the evils of society. If you hold on to your goals, the only person who can stop you is you. If you give up your goals for a few moments of pleasure with some guys who don't have your best interests at heart, you're going to be in a world of trouble. You may well ruin your life. Once you lose sight of your goals, it's going to be hard to regain them.

I know peer pressure can be very difficult to ignore. When I was growing up, there were kids who did drugs. Those were the kids I stayed away from. If it meant working out by myself or going out by myself, that's what I did. I didn't want to be associated with any-body who was using drugs or even smoking cigarettes.

In high school there were guys using drugs who approached me and wanted me to try them. Some guys on my football team were involved with drugs. They had the same goal as I did, to become a professional athlete. But they didn't stick to their goal, because they let drugs get in the way. Those are the same guys who are sitting at home now, while I am playing in the NFL. They could have been there with me if they hadn't turned to drugs.

If you are a young person in high school and you have a younger brother or sister, or if some of the children in the neighborhood look up to you, then you are an example and a role model. Those kids admire you. If you have success in sports, the younger kids in your neighborhood are going to want to be like you. They're going to want to go to high school and be on the varsity. Those same kids who are in high school now want to make it to college. They want to be like you. Some of the kids in my neighborhood said, "I want to be like Carl, he got a football scholarship to Michigan State." The sport and the school aren't important. What is important is setting a goal to get there and trying your best to reach it.

Once I got to the pros, those same kids wanted to be professionals. And another generation of kids will look up to me, just as the youngsters in the neighborhood will admire you if you are on the high school team. The importance of setting a good example starts right there in your neighborhood.

In the NFL, most of the players look unkindly on the few players who use drugs. When a player sees a teammate on drugs, or he looks around the league and sees another player using drugs such as cocaine, the first thing he wants to do is see that that guy gets help. That's what he can hope for, that that person gets help.

If the guy is a distraction or a disruptive force on the team off the field, the other players are going to insist he get some help. Your first wish is always for a player to get better, whether he's a teammate you see every day or a player on another team you've hardly even heard of. And your concern is not based on having him recover so he can help his team win. You are genuinely worried about him as a person. Life goes on after sports. None of us can play forever.

If a player is causing problems on the team, players know it's just a matter of time before he gets caught. Because if the players see it, the coaches see it and the trainers see it.

When I speak to large groups of youngsters at a school or camp, I am always asked about drugs. They ask me if I have taken drugs, if I know any players who are on drugs, how would I feel if somebody offered me drugs. It's amazing, because they sometimes seem to know more about drugs than I do. That's very sad and very scary, because a lot of these kids aren't even ten years old.

I am always honest and straightforward when I address youngsters. If they ask me a question I give them an honest answer, because I want them to know the truth. Sometimes they ask me about other players. I answer truthfully, but never do I want to ridicule a teammate, someone I have to work with. But I can't lie to those kids, because they've put their trust in me.

If someone I know is hooked on drugs, my number one wish is

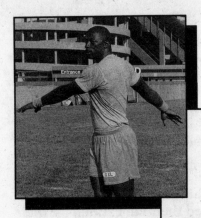

Ignore peer pressure from people who take drugs.

that he gets better. Drugs immediately moves from a football matter to a problem that affects his whole life. What a guy does on the field is important, but if you care about a teammate or a person, you want to see him get his life straightened out first.

Drugs can cost you an education and a chance at a better life.

Don't take drugs. There is so much more to life than what may be a quick moment of pleasure that you have to quickly pay to replace.

A healthy body and a healthy mind go hand-in-hand. Cleaner thoughts give you crisper motion.

Just say no. You hear it all the time on television and read it on billboards and in newspapers and it is the best advice you will ever hear. Always say no to drugs.

The most disappointing and nerve-wracking experience I had in college was due to drugs. I was a sophomore at Michigan State and I was aware that some players on the team were drug users. They were upperclassmen and some of them were starters. We had a pre-game meal in a campus hotel before home games and two hours before a game, I smelled pot in the hallway. I knew whose room it was coming from. It made me very uncomfortable, because I knew I would be on the field with guys who were strung out.

They made a lot of mistakes that game. I've seen players on a football field who were obviously on drugs and I was scared for them. They put themselves in a life-threatening situation. And they let their teammates down, because it is impossible to play as well when you are a drug user. You're not as aware of your surroundings, which is critical in football.

The following year I was one of the team captains and we had a similar incident on the road. I knew that if I went to the coaches, some of the guys on the team would lose their scholarships. They would never complete their education and some potential pro careers would never even get to training camp. But one of the assistant coaches thought he knew which players were involved, and the head coach, Muddy Waters, was ready to kick them out of school. I pleaded with Muddy for two hours to keep them. I felt bad defending two guys I knew were guilty.

But I knew if they were kicked off the team they would wind up like some of my former high school teammates, whose lives were destroyed by drugs. They had jeopardized their education and their future for the sake of marijuana, but I thought they deserved a second chance.

Those players at Michigan State begged me to get the coach to keep them on the team. I guaranteed Muddy that it wouldn't happen again. He kept them on the team, and it didn't, as far as I know. One of those players was drafted and played in the NFL.

If I add up all of my speaking engagements for a given year, I speak to about 20,000 youngsters annually. Above all else, I tell them to be good people. That may sound simplistic, but it can get you a heck of a lot further than being a bad person will.

Nobody has the good guy market cornered. Society can always use one more good person. Be yourself. Be a good person. Stay out of trouble. If you look for trouble you are going to find it. To me, the important things in being a good person are staying away from drugs and staying away from crime and getting an education to improve your life. Make your parents, other relatives, and your friends proud of you.

It doesn't require a special kind of person to do that. To be a good person doesn't take any special skills. It just takes staying out of trouble and staying away from drugs.

In today's society, a kid has two ways to go. He or she is either good or bad. There is no in between. There's also no borderline. If you are a good guy part of the time, but a bad guy at other times, then you are a bad guy. You are doing something bad or causing some kind of trouble, and that's bad. You are bad to society, and that's not good.

The talent in linebackers the year I came out (1984) was tremendous. I never thought of myself as the top linebacker eligible for the draft that year. But George Perles, who became my coach at Michi-

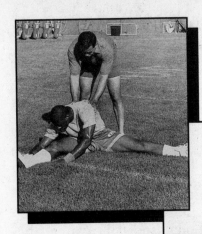

gan State after Muddy Waters had left, had been an assistant coach on the great Pittsburgh Steelers teams in the 1970s and explained a few things to me. He told me what professional scouts and coaches are looking for. Coach Perles told me that when they are looking at two or more players with almost equal ability, the first thing they do is find out what kind of person each one is. They ask themselves, will he be an asset to our team or a liability?

If a player has a bundle of talent, but is apt to hurt the team off the field because of drugs or a tendency to get in trouble, he won't be drafted as high or at all. They want tough, skilled, determined players who are also good guys. A lot of teams won't take chances on a bad guy, somebody who could well wind up being more trouble than even a lot of talent is worth. Teams are looking much more carefully now at the character of the players they are thinking of drafting.

They want a player who is going to represent himself and his team well. I never thought of myself as being the best linebacker coming out that year, because there was an abundance of talent. Many of them are still playing in the league. But I tried to do things correctly. I tried to be a good person. It paid off, because I was the third player picked in the first round.

All it took was living a clean life, getting myself in condition, and being a good person. I didn't cause a lot of problems. There are unavoidable occurrences in everyone's life. But don't go looking for trouble. Be cooperative with people you should be cooperative with. If you are a good person, people will respect you, as long as you respect yourself. You respect yourself by being a good person and doing things that are right. It rubs off onto others.

The same thing happens when you're a professional. Just like a pro athlete is a role model for youngsters, he can set an example for his teammates. How you conduct yourself off the field can rub off on the players you go into battle with. Every day in society, whether it's on a professional sports team, in an office, or in an informal gathering, people look for leaders. You are going to be either a follower or a leader. Be a leader.

You don't have to be a vocal leader. But people will look at you and they can tell whether or not they want to be like you or do some of the things you do. Even in professional sports, guys can be influenced. A perfect example is a rookie coming out of college. He needs someone to look up to when he enters the league. If there's nothing but bad examples on the team, that's what the rookie is going to relate to.

I try to extend myself to rookies. I let them know I am there to help them—whether it's coping with the adjustment to pro ball, finding a place to live, or suggesting a restaurant in Manhattan—if they want to ask me. If a young player is having trouble learning our defense, I will be more than happy to help him. I have always tried to make myself available to help my teammates. It is something I have taken even more seriously since my teammates elected me one of the Giants' captains prior to the 1989 season.

Many times, you'll see young players who are contending for your position. I never hesitate to offer them assistance. It's for the good of the team that they learn everything as well as they can, so if they ask me a question, I give them a truthful answer. By helping a teammate learn the defense, that's not going to give your job away. You keep or lose your job according to how well or how poorly you play. And the way that you play is directly affected by the way you prepare yourself. That includes both your physical state and your mental state.

When Johnie Cooks, who happens to be an outside linebacker, was traded to the Giants from the Indianapolis Colts early in the 1988 season, I helped him get comfortable in a new area and offered any assistance I could. To me, that's part of being a teammate, of being a good person.

The world is full of bad guys. You don't have to look far to find one. But a good guy is someone that's needed. Be a good guy.